Understanding
Irritable Bowel
Syndrome

Understanding Illness and Health

Many health problems and worries are strongly influenced by our thoughts and feelings. These exciting new books, written by experts in the psychology of health, are essential reading for sufferers, their families and friends.

Each book presents objective, easily understood information and advice about what the problem is, the treatments available and, most importantly, how your state of mind can help or hinder the way you cope. You will discover how to have a positive, hopeful outlook, which will help you choose the most effective treatment for you and your particular lifestyle, with confidence.

The series is edited by JANE OGDEN, Reader in Health Psychology, Guy's, King's and St Thomas' School of Medicine, King's College London, UK

Titles in the series

Understanding Irritable Bowel Syndrome

SIMON DARNLEY AND BARBARA MILLAR

WILEY

Copyright © 2003   John Wiley & Sons Ltd, The Atrium, Southern Gate, Chichester,
                     West Sussex PO19 8SQ, England

                     Telephone (+44) 1243 779777

Email (for orders and customer service enquiries): cs-books@wiley.co.uk
Visit our Home Page on www.wileyeurope.com or www.wiley.com

Reprinted May 2003

This publication is designed to provide accurate and authoritative information in regard to the subject
matter covered. It is sold on the understanding that the Publisher is not engaged in rendering
professional services. If professional advice or other expert assistance is required, the services of a
competent professional should be sought.

Other Wiley Editorial Offices

John Wiley & Sons Inc., 111 River Street, Hoboken, NJ 07030, USA

Jossey-Bass, 989 Market Street, San Francisco, CA 94103-1741, USA

Wiley-VCH Verlag GmbH, Boschstr. 12, D-69469 Weinheim, Germany

John Wiley & Sons Australia Ltd, 33 Park Road, Milton, Queensland 4064, Australia

John Wiley & Sons (Asia) Pte Ltd, 2 Clementi Loop #02-01, Jin Xing Distripark, Singapore 129809

John Wiley & Sons Canada Ltd, 22 Worcester Road, Etobicoke, Ontario, Canada M9W 1L1

Wiley also publishes its books in a variety of electronic formats. Some content that appears
in print may not be available in electronic books.

Library of Congress Cataloging-in-Publication Data

Darnley, Simon.
   Understanding irritable bowel Syndrome / Simon Darnley and Barbara Millar.
      p. cm.
Includes bibliographical references and index.
   ISBN 0-470-84496-5
1.   Irritable colon – Popular works.   I. Millar, Barbara. II. Title.

   RC862.I77 D37 2003
   616.3'42 – dc21

                                                        2002156447

British Library Cataloguing in Publication Data

A catalogue record for this book is available from the British Library

ISBN 0-470-84496-5

Contents

About the authors

SIMON DARNLEY originally qualified as a psychiatric nurse before training as a cognitive behavioural therapist. He has over 15 years experience and was tutor for the nurse cognitive behavioural training at the Institute of Psychiatry for over 6 years before coordinating and supervising a large research trial in IBS. He has developed a psychological approach to IBS that has been effective for many people. He is also a part-time magician and father of two and would like it known that while writing the book he developed many of the symptoms of IBS.

BARBARA MILLAR is a freelance journalist who has specialised in health and health services for 16 years. She has worked regularly for the *Health Service Journal*, *Nursing Times*, *Therapy Weekly* and *Health Development Today* (the magazine of the Health Development Agency), as well as writing articles for the *Times Educational Supplement*, the *Daily Mail*, *The Guardian*, *New Statesman* and *Society*. She is also a qualified Blue Badge tour guide for Scotland.

Acknowledgements

Many thanks to Bunty, Trix, Sheila (Space Mountain) and Linz; as well as to Trudie, Tom and Rodger. But most of all, thanks to Suzanne for all the support and love.

What is irritable bowel syndrome?

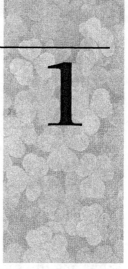

There is no simple test for irritable bowel syndrome. This chapter focuses on the symptoms that can lead to irritable bowel syndrome being diagnosed.

I am at a party making polite conversation with someone I've never met before; they ask what I do and I tell them I work in the field of IBS. Once the inevitable jokes are out of the way, I guarantee that they will either have it themselves or know someone who does. I've started to tell people I'm a train driver.

Here is Joanna's story. It's typical of the people I meet and treat with irritable bowel syndrome.

> **"**Well I think it really started when I got 'Montezuma's revenge' on holiday in the Canary Islands about 6 years ago.
>
> I was only 19 and it was my first real holiday without the parents. After that my bowel movements have never really returned to normal, I mean they are always fairly loose and runny, if you know what I mean!
>
> But the thing I hate most is the bloating, I think I retain water really easily. Since then it comes and goes but I think overall it's getting worse.
>
> It's embarrassing and often gets me down.
>
> I did go to my doctor about 2 years ago and she did various blood tests but they could not find anything.
>
> Lucy (a close friend) told me it might be a food allergy and so I cut out all wheat for a while but apart from losing a couple of pounds ... it didn't seem to help that much with the bloating or going to the toilet.**"**

Joanna's story highlights many of the key features that make up irritable bowel syndrome (we will call it IBS from now on).

If you were to ask 100 specialists from 10 countries for a definition of IBS (say for the television programme *Family Fortunes*) you would find significant differences between them. Ask them again 10 years later and, as well as the differences between them, many answers will have changed. This is because we are still learning exactly what IBS is and how best to identify it. At present it is a condition identified by the symptoms. These symptoms include pain, bloating or discomfort in the abdomen and a mixture of diarrhoea and constipation. In IBS people will experience these symptoms but we have yet to find any disease or abnormality in the body to explain it.

We know IBS is very common. In industrialised countries it affects around one in six of us. That's about a dozen people in every street!

IBS will affect people in vastly different ways. Some people will only occasionally experience symptoms, while for others the pain, diarrhoea and constipation are so severe that it becomes distressing, and affects many areas of life. It is not life-threatening, but there are times it can feel like it!

What are the signs and symptoms of IBS?

Box 1. The four main symptoms of IBS.
1. Abdominal pains: stomach pains.
2. Bloating: stomach swelling or a feeling that your stomach is bloated.
3. Diarrhoea.
4. Constipation.

There are four main symptoms of IBS, abdominal pain, diarrhoea, constipation and bloating. Other symptoms frequently found include mucus stools, increased wind, nausea and belching.

These symptoms can vary in frequency and intensity from person to person and within an individual person from day-to-day, and from month to month. Not knowing what will happen tomorrow is part of the frustrating nature of IBS:

> **"**One day it's diarrhoea and the next I can't go at all, it's the stomach pain that's the worse thing.**"**

> **"**I can go to the loo up to 40 times in one day, the next day I may not go at all, it can really get me down.**"**

> **"**When I wake up I think, 'Will I have a fat day or a thin day?'**"**

Let's look at the symptoms in more detail.

1. Pain in the abdomen

For many people abdominal pains are the most unpleasant symptom. People describe the pain in different ways; it is frequently described as coming in spasms (spasmodic); it may be nagging, sharp, heavy or dull:

> ❝I get waves of intense pain. It feels a bit like trapped wind.❞

It can be felt anywhere in the abdominal area (just below the stomach) but is more frequent down the left-hand side. The severity of this pain is the one thing most likely to drive people into seeing a doctor. Some people will describe them as 'stomach pains' even though these pains tend to occur in the abdomen:

> ❝Sometimes I'm in so much pain that I can't even sit on the toilet.❞

> ❝It feels like I have been cut in two.❞

> ❝I can cope with the diarrhoea, but the pain wears me down.❞

People may worry about what the pain may mean:

> ❝The cramps can be so bad it can't just be IBS, it must be something more serious.❞

But other people will not experience pain but rather a 'discomfort':

> ❝It's not that painful, but it is a nagging feeling.❞

Some women have found that the pains are worse prior to and during menstruation:

> ❝I just know it's going to be worse with my periods.❞

Abdominal pain is often but not always relieved by passing a stool or passing wind.

2. Bloating

Bloating or abdominal distension is common and, although for most people it is not the most severe aspect of IBS, it can be embarrassing and a nuisance:

> ❝My stomach sticks out so far that it looks like I'm pregnant. It is so embarrassing.❞

> ❝I spend most of my time in tracksuits to cover it up.❞

> ❝My boyfriend wants to go out all the time and I have to make excuses as I don't want to go out when I'm bloated.❞

> ❝It makes me feel ugly.❞

> ❝I swear sometimes I can see it growing.❞

When people have been asked about bloating, they describe a very similar pattern. People find that the mornings are generally good but their abdomens will gradually distend or bloat throughout the day. By the evenings the bloating can become so bad that tight clothes such as jeans no longer fit.

Some people also find that eating will bring on the bloating:

> ❝I know eating at lunchtime will bring on the bloating, so if I have to go out in the evening I will skip lunch altogether.❞

Others swear that specific foods are responsible:

> ❝I know it sounds weird but fruit, especially bananas, seems to make the bloating worse.❞

Some doctors were unsure whether the bloating was a 'real symptom' and there was an increase in waist size or whether it was a subjective feeling in that people felt tightness but there was no actual waist expansion. It has now been demonstrated that bloating is associated with an increase in waist size and that this would gradually increase throughout the day, sometimes up to 4 inches!

Abdominal bloating is associated with discomfort, increased wind (flatulence) and rumbling noises (borborygmi):

> ❝I try and avoid meetings at work–I worry that I will pass wind, it really smells bad, it would be so embarrassing.❞

> ❝If I relax the wind can be really disgusting ... I avoid sex wherever possible.❞

3. Diarrhoea

We have all had diarrhoea at some point in our lives. When our stools are very runny, mushy or watery we know we have diarrhoea. Its one of those words which, along with constipation, everyone understands but is hard to define.

> ❝I thought the world had exploded out of my bottom.❞

This is recognised as an episode/attack or bout of diarrhoea. Commonly, but not necessarily exclusively, this attack of diarrhoea will be associated with wanting to use the toilet immediately and more frequently than normal. The urge to go can be very strong and sometimes painful:

> ❝I knew I had to go and I had to go then!❞

> ❝There was no warning, I just had to drop everything and go!❞

> ❝The feeling was overwhelming, I was so worried I would not make it [to the toilet].❞

Some people will experience normal stools at the beginning of the day followed by very loose watery stools, and then regular stools for the rest of the day:

> ❝I can have what I call normal and runny stools in a matter of hours!❞

Others will experience an increased bout of going to the toilet but do not pass watery stools; instead they may pass frequent solid stools:

> ❝I go up to 15 times in a morning, but each time I will pass a fairly solid stool.❞

This is not diarrhoea. It is still a very common symptom in IBS but different to diarrhoea as the stools are not watery. Some experts have named this phenomenon 'pseudodiarrhoea'.

4. Constipation

As we have seen with diarrhoea, constipation can be difficult to define but most people will understand what it is:

> ❝I pass very small rabbit poos.❞

> ❝I only go about once or twice a week if I'm lucky, and even then it's very hard and lumpy.❞

The main features are small hard lumpy stools and infrequent defecation.

But we know some people have always tended to pass infrequent hard lumpy stools and do not see themselves as constipated; for them that is normal. It may be that they are constipated but they do not know they are and manage to live their lives quite happily without suffering any other symptoms.

In IBS, constipation is often associated with straining, or a feeling you want to go but can't:

> ❝I will sit and strain for up to 30 minutes sometimes. If I'm lucky I'll pass a small amount.❞

> ❝I often feel I want to go quite desperately, but when I try and go nothing comes out.❞

> ❝It can be very difficult to go!❞

Some people have tried to define constipation as occurring when people go less than three times a week. Generally this is a reasonable guide, but it's not definitive. Some people who may go three times one week and four times the next are very likely to still suffer from constipation.

In IBS constipation can be mixed up with the other symptoms:

> ❝I can pass small painful stools in the morning and then normal ones in the evening!❞

Some people with IBS may pass small, hard, lumpy stools several times a day and believe they have diarrhoea, where in fact they will have constipation.

Symptoms associated with IBS

1. Mucus stools

The passage of mucus with stools is a fairly common symptom in IBS. People who experience this will describe slimy or watery stools:

> ❝It's like jelly but not quite set!❞

It tends to occur more often in patients who experience more constipation and sometimes the mucus stools can be misinterpreted as runny, diarrhoea-type stools.

2. A feeling of incomplete evacuation

> ❝Take yesterday, I had just passed a large stool and yet it still felt there was something left to come out!❞

> ❝Most days I feel I should go, even if I have been recently . . . But when I try nothing comes out.❞

❝It's a feeling like you want to go to the toilet but you can't, it feels trapped in my guts!❞

This feeling is common in IBS. Doctors call it a 'feeling of incomplete evacuation'. This sensation is a very common symptom associated with IBS. It often leads to a constant awareness of the rectal area and excessive straining:

❝I seem to be constantly aware that my bowel is never empty.❞

❝I will strain for up to 30 minutes every time I go.❞

❝I can feel it's there, I strain for ages but I can't pass anything.❞

It should not be confused with tenesmus which is a painful and violent urge to pass a stool. This rarely occurs in IBS

3. Urgency and incontinence

I'm sure we have all experienced an urgent sense that we have to go to the toilet immediately. With IBS this is a regular feature, along with diarrhoea. Although many people worry they will not make it in time and become incontinent, our research has found this is, thankfully, rare. However, another study suggested that 16 per cent of IBS sufferers have experienced bowel incontinence at some time or another.

4. Wind

The average woman will passes wind 12 times per day, and the average man will pass wind 18 times per day. People with IBS frequently pass more wind than the average person, have more awareness of it and will worry more about the embarrassment it may cause:

❝When I have a bout of IBS, my wind can be disgusting, I really worry about letting one go in front of people at work. I have called in sick if it's too bad.❞

❝I don't like it when I relax in company as I know I am more likely to break wind.❞

5. Nausea, vomiting and belching

Nausea is an uncomfortable feeling in the stomach that is usually accompanied by the urge to vomit. Although not common in IBS, some people do experience these symptoms as part of their IBS.

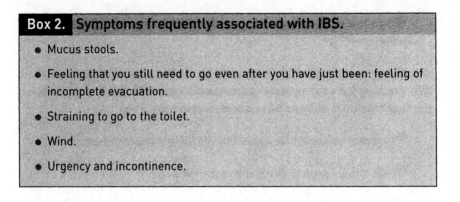

Box 2. Symptoms frequently associated with IBS.

- Mucus stools.
- Feeling that you still need to go even after you have just been: feeling of incomplete evacuation.
- Straining to go to the toilet.
- Wind.
- Urgency and incontinence.

People with IBS can also have other symptoms not related to the bowels. These include: nausea, belching, vomiting, feeling full after eating only a small meals, tiredness, problems with passing water (urinating) and pain during intercourse.

Defining IBS

We have described many of the symptoms that make up IBS, but how do doctors then diagnose the problem? If you were expecting to find a clear definition of IBS in this section you may be disappointed. We have already said there is no definitive medical test that a doctor can give people to verify whether they have IBS. This makes IBS a clinical diagnosis. The doctor will make a diagnosis based on the symptoms a patient has over a period of time. He or she will check the person does not have any symptoms that would indicate other illnesses and only proceed with the diagnosis once these have been ruled out. For example, in younger people a doctor would want to rule out the possibility of inflammatory bowel disease, and in older people (50+) he or she would want to check for the possibility of colorectal cancer (see Chapter 2 on seeing a doctor). Only after checking this out would the doctor then make a diagnosis of IBS. It can sometimes be difficult to recognise and doctors and patients can be uncertain whether they actually have it or not. Symptoms usually fluctuate and may not occur for months or even years, or the person may find it hard to describe all their symptoms.

Over the years experts have worked to develop and refine criteria that will help make it easier to diagnose IBS. Having a recognisable set of criteria in diagnosing IBS has many advantages. Diagnoses can be transferable to other health professionals and insurance companies, ensuring some consistency between all those working in the field around the world.

The first attempt at developing specific criteria for IBS was published in 1978. Researchers at Bristol derived the Manning criteria (named after the main researcher) from symptoms reported by patients with abdominal pain who attended a hospital gastroenterology department. They found that six symptoms were more prevalent in IBS than in other organic diseases. These criteria were then tested and validated in a community setting.

Box 3.	The six symptoms in the manning criteria of IBS.

1. Visible abdominal distension.

2. Relief of pain with bowel movement.

3. More frequent bowel movement with the onset of pain.

4. Loose stools at the onset of pain.

5. Passage of mucus per rectum.

6. Feeling of incomplete evacuation.

Manning studied the differences between organic disease and IBS in patients attending his gastroenterology clinic on the basis of the symptoms they described. The study was performed on 109 patients and only 32 were diagnosed with IBS after about two years.

The Manning criteria have since been validated by others around the world and shown to be able to differentiate IBS from organic gastrointestinal disease.

It is suggested that symptoms should be present for at least 3 months in the current year to rule out other problems.

The Rome criteria

An international group of gastroenterologists with a special interest in IBS felt that, while the Manning criteria were a good start, they needed refining. A set of criteria was needed that was more specific and useful when conducting research in IBS. To try and come up with a universal definition of IBS, a conference was held in Rome in 1988. The top experts in the field from Europe and North America gathered, discussed and agreed on their own criteria, which became known as the 'Rome I criteria of IBS'. The Rome criteria were promoted for use in IBS epidemiological studies and as entry criteria for clinical trials.

A couple of years later the experts returned to Rome to further refine the criteria (Rome II; Thompson *et al.*, 1999). Some specialists and doctors thought that, although the Rome II provided clear criteria for clinical research in IBS, it was too restrictive. One study suggested that, using the Rome II criteria, about two-thirds of patients diagnosed with IBS by the Rome I criteria would be excluded. Whether the Rome II criteria were too restrictive or the Rome I criteria were too lax was the talk of many gastroenterologists.

So they all went to Rome again and agreed on Rome III. Rome III is not so rigid as Rome II and, in addition to the criteria for IBS, the consensus group also gave advice concerning the investigations necessary to exclude organic disease. The Rome III criteria should be published in 2003.

Box 4. Rome III criteria for IBS.

At least 12 weeks, which need to be consecutive, in the preceding 12 months of abdominal discomfort or pain that has two of three features:

(1) relieved by defecation; and/or

(2) onset associated with a change in frequency of stool; and/or

(3) onset associated with a change in form (appearance) of stool.

The following symptoms cumulatively support the diagnosis of IBS

- Abnormal stool frequency (>3/day and <3/week) (more than three times a day and less than three times a week).

- Abnormal stool form (lumpy/hard or loose/watery stool.)

- Abnormal stool passage (straining, urgency, or feeling of incomplete evacuation).

- Passage of mucus.

- Bloating or feeling of abdominal distension.

The Kruis criteria (1984)

The Kruis criteria never really took off and are not widely used. I'm only including them in this section for the sake of completeness. Kruis understood that IBS is difficult to diagnose and he believed that many people may be diagnosed with IBS when they actually have something else (we call this a false positive). Kruis tried to define criteria for IBS that would reduce this risk of overlooking an organic disease. If a person meets his criteria then they should indicate IBS with a positive predictive value of 94 per cent.

Box 5.	The Kruis diagnostic criteria.

	Score
A. Questions to be completed by the patient	

1. Are you here because of abdominal pain?
   Do you suffer from flatulence?
   Do you suffer from irregular bowel movements?
	+34

2. Have you suffered from your complaints for more than two years?	+16

3. How can your abdominal pain be described – burning,
   cutting, very strong, terrible, feeling of pressure, dull,
   boring, not so bad?
	+23

4. Have you noticed alternating constipation and diarrhoea?	+14
B. Checklist to be completed by the Doctor	
1. Abnormal physical findings and/or history pathogenic for any diagnosis other than IBS	−47
2. ESR > 20 mm/2 hours	−13
3. Leukocytosis >10 000/cm	−50
4. Haemoglobin: female <12 g per cent, male <14 g per cent	−98
5. History of blood in stool	−98

A score of 44 or more indicates IBS with a predictive value of 94 per cent.

IBS sub-types

Some doctors will break down their patients with IBS into sub-types, labelling people as diarrhoea-predominant IBS or constipation-predominant IBS. Drug companies are especially keen on trying to identify different sub-types of IBS. This is because they can then target their drugs to helping constipation or diarrhoea specifically. Of course, as we have already mentioned, many people alternate between the two conditions and it can be difficult to categorise IBS in this way.

A concise history of IBS

IBS has been described as far back as the nineteenth century. Of course it was not called irritable bowel syndrome back then. Early accounts placed more emphasis on the discharge of mucus from the rectum; this seems a much rarer symptom today. IBS has been known by many names – colitis, mucous colitis, spastic colon, spastic bowel, and functional bowel disease. None of these terms accurately describe IBS. Colitis, for example, means inflammation of the large intestine (colon); but we know IBS does not cause inflammation. Dolhart was the first to coin the term 'Irritable bowel syndrome' in 1946. The name has been widely accepted, mainly because it is so vague and non-specific. The word 'syndrome' also suggests multiple symptoms. It does not mention the part of the bowel that is irritable or why it is irritable. In 1962 Dr Chaudhary published a paper called 'The irritable colon syndrome' (Chaudhary and Truelove, 1962). This was the first systematic review on the condition. It was later discovered that more than the colon was involved and the name developed to 'irritable bowel'. Around Europe IBS may be called 'Reizdarm', 'colica mucosa', 'colitis spastica', 'colon irritable' and 'prikkelbare darm' syndrome.

How common is IBS?

We can see how the prevalence of IBS will vary considerably, depending on the diagnostic criteria used; but, despite this, it is very common (around 15 per cent in Western countries). If you don't suffer from it yourself then I'm pretty sure you know someone who does. Studies of the prevalence of IBS have shown substantial differences between different countries (see Box 6).

The differences may be partly due to the different ways of defining IBS. In Denmark the prevalence of IBS was found to be 5–65 per cent, depending on the definition of IBS used, but this can't explain all the differences. Other factors such as the ethnic mix may also affect the prevalence of IBS. In one American study IBS was five times more prevalent in white populations than in black populations. There may be other factors that affect prevalence, such as economic and social changes. Two studies looking at the incidence of IBS in Africa 11 years apart found conflicting and interesting results. The first study in 1984 suggested that IBS was rare in native Africans. In 1995 IBS was found to be around 30 per cent among the native population. In the intervening 11 years there have been significant economic and social changes in the areas studied. Could these affect the incidence of IBS?

Box 6.	IBS around the world.

France	13%
Netherlands	9%
Sweden	13%
New Zealand	16%
USA	15%
UK	14%
Brazil	9%
Denmark	65%*
China	23%
Japan	25%
Singapore	3%
Iran	3%
Nigeria	30%

*Different diagnostic criteria for IBS used.

Who is more likely to get IBS?

Nearly half the people with IBS will have symptoms before the age of 30. Generally women are affected by IBS far more than men. About 75 per cent of people with IBS are women. Not only are women more likely to have IBS, but also they are more likely to visit their doctor than men. This means that in some medical centres women make up over 90 per cent of people with IBS. It may be that cultural factors are also important. For example, in India and Sri Lanka it was found that men were more likely to report IBS than women (26 per cent women to 74 per cent men)

The course of IBS

The occurrence of IBS seems to decrease the older we get. No one is quite sure why. It has been suggested that this may be related to changes in the gut; or maybe it's just that older people don't report the symptoms so often – we are still unsure.

What are the prospects for IBS?

IBS is a chronic condition. That means that once you get it, it's likely to stay with you for many years. The good news is the symptoms will vary over time, so between the bouts of symptoms you will also have periods with minimal symptoms or no symptoms at all.

When a number of people were asked about their symptoms a year or more apart, some people who had the symptoms had lost them. At the same time roughly an equal number of people who did not have symptoms had acquired them. The proportion of people with IBS is still roughly the same at around 15 per cent, but the people making up this 15 per cent will change from year to year.

Is it harmful?

NO!

Most people with IBS believe at some point during the illness that there is something seriously wrong with their gut. It can feel like that! IBS is often painful, uncomfortable and inconvenient and can cause a great deal of discomfort and distress, but it does not cause permanent harm to the intestines. There is no indication that there is any physical damage that occurs to people suffering from IBS. It does not lead to intestinal bleeding of the bowel or to a serious disease such as cancer, inflammatory bowel disease or Crohn's disease. As one expert put it:

> **"**Comfortingly few have developed gut disease and, in those that do, the disease is benign and unrelated to the original symptoms.**"**

Summary

- Irritable bowel syndrome is a common disorder of the intestines that leads to pain, bloating and changes in bowel habits (diarrhoea and/or constipation).

- There is no current test available to identify IBS. It is diagnosed from the symptoms and by ruling out organic problems.

- Consensual criteria have been developed to help diagnose IBS.

- IBS generally occurs before the age of 30 and affects twice as many women as men.

- IBS is a chronic condition but the nature and severity of the symptoms will vary widely between people and may also change over time in the individual.

- Although often painful and inconvenient, IBS is not known to harm people suffering from it.

Causes and effects of IBS

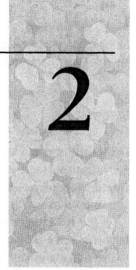

In this chapter we examine the various theories suggested to explain the cause of IBS. If you think there are problems in trying to define IBS, just wait until you read about the problems of trying to work out what is behind IBS.

There are many possible causes and effects of IBS. Some causes are psychological, such as stress, and some are physiological, including theories of gut motility. Many people complain that their doctors just don't take their symptoms seriously, and that some go so far as to say that they are all in the mind. Describing a symptom as being psychological is seen as being dismissive. We do know that all symptoms will get worse if you focus on them and will get better if you are distracted. IBS symptoms are no different.

CASE STUDY CASE STUDY CASE STUDY CASE STUDY

Lindsey's IBS was in full swing. Her stomach was bloated and painful. She had to go to an appointment with her son's teacher to discuss his progress. Because of her IBS, she really wanted to miss it, but knew it would be a long time before she got another chance to discuss Jack's progress so forced herself to go. After discussing Jack with the teacher she bumped into an old friend who was also at the school to discuss Joanna, her daughter. They went for a drink together and when Lindsey returned some hours later her husband Tom enquired about her IBS. Lindsey told him that although her stomach was still bloated she really had not noticed the pain until he had just then mentioned it.

Therefore, we think that the best way to understand any symptom is as a combination of psychological and physiological factors. These psychological and physiological factors are described below.

Causes

I have worked with many general practitioners (GPs), psychologists, psychiatrists, psychotherapists and gastroenterologists, mostly experts in their field, who have treated many people with IBS. When asked what they think causes IBS, they all answer in different ways, depending on their own background and training.

It has been suggested that IBS should be called 'intestinal symptoms, cause unknown' as it highlights our current lack of understanding of what IBS is all about.

Let's try and piece together all the various arguments and evidence around the cause of IBS in an attempt to make sense of it all.

The role of what we eat

Many people are aware that they are sensitive to certain foods and know that if they have too much of them they will 'suffer for it' later on:

> **"**I guarantee that if I have a curry and six pints I will very likely have diarrhoea the next day.**"**

Many people claim that IBS is caused by food intolerances and allergies. This is not the case and there is very little convincing evidence that it is the case (for more further details see Chapter 3). This is very common and not surprising. We know that when people have IBS, food intolerances tend to increase as the intestines become more sensitive. Also intolerances that were fairly minor may become more of a problem.

This suggests that food intolerances are a *result* of IBS and not the cause.

Many alternative therapists and dietitians may claim that one of the causes of IBS is what we eat (see Chapter 3 on diet and Chapter 6 on alternative treatments for more details). On the face of it, this claim does appear to have some plausibility. People with IBS see what they put in their mouths at one end coming out as diarrhoea or constipation at the other, and they also associate this with the pain and bloating they experience, but no research has yet clearly demonstrated this to be the case.

When constipation is induced in normal volunteers they develop symptoms of IBS. As a lack of fibre can cause constipation, some people have suggested that a reduction of fibre in the diet may also cause IBS. But when researchers examined the amount of fibre eaten in the daily diets of people with IBS and in the diets of people without IBS, they found that both groups were eating a similar amount. So it is unlikely that IBS is due to a lack of fibre.

Many people claim to be intolerant of certain foods. They know that eating these foods will cause IBS. In our experience these foods are many and varied and often quite individual in nature:

> ❝Orange juice will cause the runs, but apple juice is OK.❞

> ❝I can eat tomatoes when cooked but only raw without the skins.❞

Food intolerances are quite hard to prove objectively. Many people associate one bad experience with a certain food and then promptly remove it from their diet. Often they do not check out whether this was, indeed, the food that caused the increase in IBS symptoms. We know that the very act of eating can induce bowel symptoms. This can be in a non-specific way or as a result of large meals, irregular meals, eating too quickly or binge eating.

Many people with IBS claim to be allergic to certain foods. A recent study suggested that nearly one in ten of us claim to have some food allergy but, when tested, only two in every hundred actually do.

The role of the movement of stools through our guts

Some experts used to think IBS was due to abnormalities in the process of the movement of stools through the digestive system. Doctors call this a *motility disorder*. On the surface this makes some sense, as most people with IBS do, at some time, have either constipation or diarrhoea and so stools pass through the system either slowly or very rapidly. Studies have shown abnormal electrical activity in people with IBS.

The role of the nervous system

> ❝The fault lies in the nervous control of the intestine rather than in the intestine itself.❞

Recently an increasing amount of research has been conducted on the enteric nervous system (ENS) and its role in the cause of IBS. The ENS is a large bundle of nerves found in the wall of the intestine. It contains as many nerves as the spinal cord and is often called the 'gut brain'. The gut is linked to the ENS and the ENS has links with the central nervous system (CNS). Pathways from the brain have been shown to modify or make changes in the activity of the pathways from the gut. Some people suggest that this is why our moods and emotions have such an effect on the symptoms of IBS.

Michael Gershon, a senior American anatomist and cell biologist explains:

> **❝**Nerve transmissions between the brain and the nerves lining the walls of the intestines mean that the mind and the gut 'talk' to one another. The brain sends signals to the digestive system and influences activity there. The reverse is also true – any distress felt in the bowels can also cause mental distress.**❞**

Researchers suggest that by studying the chemistry and make-up of the ENS they may find the answer to IBS. This study of the ENS and its connection to the CNS is called neurogastroenterology. Nothing has yet been found, but it's still early days and developments are awaited.

The gut can be such a sensitive thing

Although the cause of IBS is not yet fully understood, recent research has revealed that the bowel in IBS sufferers tends to be more sensitive than in people without IBS and this sensitivity can set off a reaction which causes the symptoms.

In a study at the University College of Los Angeles (Moore, no date), IBS people were tested by inflating balloons in their intestines and pain sensitivity levels were measured, together with the amount of tension in the muscles of the intestines before and after the balloon treatment.

If you slowly inflate a balloon in the rectum of a person with IBS they will feel the pain and discomfort at a smaller size (volume or pressure) than people without IBS. This is called visceral hypersensitivity and is currently all the rage. It seems that most people with IBS have visceral hypersensitivity.

I would like to meet the person who first thought of blowing up balloons in people's rectums. He sounds like an interesting guy!

When the same experiment was conducted in the small intestine and also in the oesophagus, the pain thresholds in people with IBS were again found to be more sensitive. But pain thresholds were the same for people both with and without IBS when skin was tested. This suggests that people with IBS have a higher sensitivity to all the gut areas but not all over the body.

Some people have criticised the idea of visceral hypersensitivity, pointing out that anyone about to have a balloon inflated in their rectum would be really focusing on that area, knowing it was going to cause pain and expecting the worst. They suggest that the 'increased sensitivity' could be down to the expectation of pain and not to an actual sensitivity of the rectum.

In order to counteract this criticism, the researchers carried out further experiments, using balloons of different sizes and sometimes not inflating the balloon at all. The results revealed that people with IBS did not feel the balloon at lower volumes than people without IBS but rather that they reported *all* sensations as unpleasant and painful. Visceral hypersensitivity could explain why people with IBS experience so much pain.

Hyposensitivity has also been shown to occur in IBS. This is the opposite case, where the gut is much *less* sensitive than in people without IBS. Hyposensitivity is generally only seen in people with constipation, especially those people who very rarely experience any urge to go at all.

There were also altered responses by both the brain and the gut to balloon inflation in the intestines. The brain responses were measured using an imaging technique called positron emission tomography (PET) and, in IBS people, the brain responded to the stresses and stimuli in the gut differently than in healthy individuals, confirming, stated the researchers, that there is a definite brain/gut connection with IBS.

The role of inflammation

Studies have recently shown that many people who recover from an inflammation, such as ulcerative colitis will go on to have IBS symptoms even after the inflammation has healed.

The role of infections

❝I got really bad food poisoning in Ibiza three years ago, I was laid out for two days ... since then things have never really returned to normal. My guts seem much more sensitive to what I eat and I have diarrhoea at least three times a week.❞

Large numbers of people describe a very similar onset to their IBS. Recent studies have shown around 25 per cent of people with IBS go on to develop it after a bout of gastroenteritis or acute gut infection. Interestingly, vomiting during the gastroenteritis seems to offer protection against the development of IBS.

Salmonella and *Campylobacter* are the most common infections but it seems that many microorganisms can cause the same reaction. Some doctors will use the term *post-infective irritable bowel syndrome (PI-IBS)*. This does not mean that bacteria are the cause of IBS but rather that the inflammation caused through the gastroenteritis – and not the infection itself – is one of the triggers that leads to IBS.

The role of emotions

❝I know that if I have an important meeting at work I will get really bad IBS in the morning.❞

Most of us realise that the state of our bowels is related to the way we think and feel. Phrases such as 'gut feeling', 'shit scared' and 'tight arsed' all suggest we commonly link our guts with the way we feel.

A study among college students and hospital employees found that 71 per cent of them reported that stress affected their bowel pattern, with 54 per cent reporting that it led to abdominal pain or discomfort. Other studies have also demonstrated the relationship between daily stress and digestive symptoms on women with or without IBS. They found a relationship between reported levels of daily stress and daily symptoms such as bloating and diarrhoea. Both groups, those with and without IBS, were affected.

In one study 65 per cent of people with IBS reported a severely stressful event prior to developing IBS. These included death of a partner or family member, starting a new job, and even a prison sentence.

Fear and panic also have a direct influence on bowel function. One study compared people who were diagnosed and seeking treatment for panic disorder and a group of individuals without any panic disorder. IBS was diagnosed in 46.3 per cent of the people with panic disorder but only 2.5 per cent of the people without panic disorder had IBS.

Psychiatric illnesses such as anxiety and depression have been found in around 40 per cent of people with IBS who are referred to a specialist. In comparison, these illnesses are only found in around 20 per cent of people with other gastrointestinal disorders. It has long been thought that people with IBS have greater psychological disturbances than people without IBS and many studies have previously reported this. However, these people with IBS represent only a small proportion of people who had been selected and referred to specialised gastroenterology units, as the majority of people with IBS are never referred to these units. This leads to an over-estimation of the degree of psychological disturbances in the IBS population.

When people with IBS who do not see their doctor are compared with those without IBS, both groups have similar levels of psychological illness. This does not mean that IBS is a psychiatric disorder, or that it is all in the mind.

This is very important. Just because there is no current identifiable structure or abnormality found in IBS does not mean that the symptoms are in a person's head. This suggests that the symptoms are somehow not real or that the person is making them up or exaggerating their severity. People who think that 'it is all in the head' are separating the mind from the body. We call this dualistic thinking – that something is either physical or mental. This is not the case and the view is based on very outdated medical ways of thinking about illness. What is important is to try to view the whole person and all the surrounding issues as important parts of IBS.

The role of anger

In a study examining the effects of anger on the colon in IBS, people with IBS were compared with people without IBS. Both groups were examined resting and during two anger situations, which consisted of criticising performance in an intelligence test and delaying help during a medical procedure.

When resting, people with IBS were observed to have more active colons than normal subjects. Anger increased colon muscle activity in both people with IBS and people without IBS, compared with the resting state. However, people with IBS produced *significantly* higher colon muscle activity when angered. They also reported themselves to be more hostile and appeared angrier than normal controls after the study. It seems that anger is another emotion able to trigger the brain–gut connection and, in the same way as stress, it will cause an increase in IBS symptoms.

Before writing this book we had to write a proposal outlining the topics we wanted to cover. This was sent to experts in the field of IBS. One reviewer wrote back:

> **❝**I strongly believe that IBS is not a psychological condition, although like just about any disease, it can, of course, be made worse by stress. The author of this proposal comes from a psychological background and this could possibly perpetuate the myth that IBS is a purely psychological condition.**❞**

Hopefully we have shown that IBS is definitely not a 'purely psychological condition' and that this does not account for the onset of IBS. However, it may be that the role psychological factors play in IBS is significant and more important than in many other gastrointestinal conditions.

Can we learn to experience IBS symptoms?

Researchers from Washington interviewed 271 children about their symptoms and found those who had parents with IBS reported more gastrointestinal (IBS-like) symptoms than children who did not have parents suffering from IBS. Children with parents with IBS were also found to miss more school for IBS-like complaints and were taken to the doctor more often.

Children whose parents have IBS have been shown to attend medical clinics more often than other children. This does suggest that the development of IBS may, in part, be due to the way we are taught to respond to symptoms. This is sometimes called illness behaviour. What did your parents do when you were ill? Mine were very strict and sent me off to school even if I really did have a stomach-ache, but some children's parents respond very differently:

> "When I was sick as a child my mum used to take time off work and look after me, we used to cuddle up on the sofa and watch daytime TV. They are amongst my happiest memories of my childhood."

> "I know I worry too much about my IBS, I'm like my mum ... she is a bit of a hypochondriac ... when I was young she used to take me to the doctors all the time."

This does not mean that parents cause IBS, but the way we respond to the symptoms of IBS does seem to play a part in the way they then develop:

> "My uncle died of cancer, and even though the doctor has told me not to worry, I can't help but think ...."

> "It's mainly constipation with me, I enjoy food but I can't get rid of it. I'm sure I'm storing up problems."

> "I think about my bowels too much."

> "I don't think it's OK to leave it in there."

A comparison of people diagnosed with IBS by a doctor and people with the same symptoms who had not consulted a doctor revealed that those who had been to the doctor not only experienced more pain but were also more concerned about serious diseases than those who did not consult.

Sexual trauma and IBS

Researchers have also examined the relationship between sexual abuse and IBS. Psychiatric and sexual trauma interviews of people with IBS and those with inflammatory bowel disease (IBD) were carried out. The frequency of sexual abuse in the two groups was then compared. The results were revealing. People with IBS had a significantly higher rate of severe sexual trauma (32 per cent versus 0 per cent) and severe childhood sexual abuse (11 per cent versus 0 per cent) compared with people with inflammatory bowel problems.

A biopsychosocial or combined model of IBS

Rather than attributing the onset of IBS to one specific cause, it is more sensible to see IBS as being caused by many factors combining together. This has been called a biopsychosocial model of IBS and suggests that physiological and emotional aspects, thoughts and behaviours are all involved in IBS. This model is further explained in the treatment chapters.

How can I be sure I have IBS and it is not something more serious?

While IBS can cause distress and discomfort it does differ from a serious disease such as bowel cancer. At first sight many of the symptoms seem to be the same and many people worry that their symptoms mean they have a more serious problem.

Ask yourselves the following questions

1. Do the symptoms usually come and go over hours or days?

   If the answer is yes, then it is more likely you have IBS. In serious disease the symptoms are usually persistent.

2. Do the symptoms vary from time to time? For example sometimes you have constipation and sometimes diarrhoea, sometimes the pain will vary in its position or vary depending on your mood and amount of stress going on in your life? Do you find if you are busy many of the symptoms are more bearable?

   Again, if you answer yes to these questions, then it is more likely you have IBS. In serious disease the symptoms tend to be stereotyped in a regular way.

3. Do the pains or bloating ease off when you open your bowels or do you have feelings you still want to pass a stool even if you have just been?

Once again, if the answer is yes to this question, then it is more likely to be IBS. Unless these symptoms are associated with being sick or bleeding then is unlikely to be any serious disease.

I also pass more urine. Does this mean something more serious? ▶

No, this is also common in IBS, the bladder can become sensitive as well as the bowel; and this is common in women and may also cause some pain during sexual intercourse.

Any single symptom of IBS can possibly be caused by a serious illness, but the large number, the variety and the fluctuating nature of symptoms experienced by sufferers of IBS tend to suggest a functional disorder and not a serious disease.

Associated conditions and symptoms

Many people with IBS also suffer from a wide variety of symptoms not associated with the bowel. Dyspeptic symptoms are most prevalent, affecting between 58 and 94 per cent of people with IBS. Females with IBS seem to have more digestive health problems and non-digestive health problems than men with IBS. Tiredness, backache, bladder and gynaecological symptoms are also common.

IBS and fibromyalgia

Fibromyalgia is an inflammation of the fibrous tissues of the skeletal system. People suffering from fibromyalgia will experience pain, extreme tiredness and sleep disturbances. Even though IBS and fibromyalgia are different disorders, a number of studies have discovered that they are often found together. In one study, 41 per cent of people with fibromyalgia also had IBS and in another study of people with IBS 68 per cent reported back pain and 70 per cent reported fatigue. Unfortunately nothing has yet been found to link the two conditions. It does not seem that IBS makes the fibromyalgia worse or vice versa.

Gynaecological aspects of IBS

Women with IBS tend to suffer from more painful periods as well as increased IBS symptoms at the time of their period. It is also common for women to experience pain on intercourse, sufficiently severe for it to affect their enjoyment of sex. This pain is often described as being very similar to their bowel pain and comes on some time after sex. This can cause a lot of stress in some relationships:

❝... I avoid sex with my husband as much as possible, it's not that I don't love him or anything, it's just that it often hurts after and my IBS then gets worse ... He doesn't understand it ... how can my IBS affect sex?**❞**

Lower abdominal pain in IBS can frequently be confused with other gynaecological problems. Nearly 50 per cent of women seeing a gynaecologist for lower abdominal pain also suffer from IBS. If you have IBS you are nearly three times more likely to have a hysterectomy than a woman who does not have IBS. This often means that many women undergo a wide variety of needless gynaecological tests, treatments and surgery without any benefit. Ironically, abdominal surgery has been shown to actually make the symptoms of IBS worse.

The effect of IBS

So far we have listed the many symptoms of IBS and the many factors that may influence its onset but the real issue is the way that IBS affects people.

IBS can have a serious effect on work:

❝I haven't worked for a couple of years now, I don't know if I could make the commitment, some days the pain and diarrhoea are so bad that I dare not stray too far from the toilet. It may only happen a couple of times a month but I don't seem to get a warning.**❞**

One survey has found that people with IBS symptoms missed three times as many workdays as other people.

Another, larger survey of American and British people with IBS found nearly a third of those asked missed at least one day of work in the last month due to IBS. Over 45 per cent cut back on work and other activities due to IBS. Taken together, the average time lost or cut back over a four-week period was five days or one working week!

It's not just missing work due to IBS symptoms, many people are much more reluctant to take promotion or job opportunities:

❝Every year the team go to head office in Holland; I would love to go but dare not risk it.**❞**

❝They have offered me promotion on a number of occasions ... I have made many excuses but the real reason is that I am not sure how my IBS would cope with the extra responsibility and commitment.**❞**

Many people with IBS are now working from home:

66Since I got a computer and can work from home it has really helped. The IBS is just as bad, but I feel more in control of it.99

IBS also has just as much effect on relationships and social life:

66When my IBS flares up, I'm totally off limits to any thing with other people.99

66I used to love the cinema but I haven't been for years.99

Areas such as physical functioning, general health, vitality, social functioning, sexual relations and mental health can all be seriously affected. The intensity of the pain seems to be significant, the worse the pain is the worse the effect IBS has on your quality of life:

66It seems to dominate me, I can't forget it for more than a few moments.99

Getting the best out of going to your doctor

If you think you have IBS you must see your doctor. This is because your doctor can rule out other more serious diseases with some similar symptoms to IBS. The typical features of IBS are recognisable by doctors. He or she will ask you to describe your symptoms, will examine your abdomen and may even take a blood test. He or she will then be able to recognise the IBS and, in most cases, rule out other medical disorders. It may be that for the majority of the time you can cope with your symptoms but, by discussing them with your doctor, you can prepare for those times when it may become difficult. Some people will put off going to the doctor for as long as possible (mostly men!). Our advice is to go early and be prepared.

Due to increasing numbers of people constantly competing for doctors' time and energy, you are likely to get anything from 4 to 10 minutes at any one appointment.

HELPFUL TIPS HELPFUL TIPS! HELPFUL TIPS! HELPFUL

How to prepare for an appointment with your doctor about IBS

Make a list of answers to these questions in preparation for the consultation. ▶

If you have pain

Is the pain always in the same place or does it move around?

How often do you get it and how long does it last?

What happens to the pain when you open your bowels?

In·what other situations are you more likely to experience pain (for example, when under stress)?

If you have bloating

How often do you experience bloating and how long does it last?

Is the visible bloating there when you wake up in the morning?

Is it worse at any particular time of day?

If you have diarrhoea and constipation

How many times do you go on a good day/bad day?

When you have been to the toilet, do you feel as if you have not completely emptied your bowels and that you could go some more if pushed?

Have you ever felt the need to go but couldn't?

Have you ever been incontinent?

Is the diarrhoea constant?

How were your bowel habits before this all started?

Other questions to answer

Have you ever noticed blood in your stools?

Have you lost a significant amount of weight recently?

What are your current medications, and allergies?

Do your best to make the brief time you have with your doctor worth the effort you put in to get there. Be inquisitive and make sure you really understand what the doctor is saying. If you have difficulty in remembering the conversation, take a tape recorder to the appointment. Any doctor worth his salt will not mind at all.

Remember: every second counts!

The majority of people with IBS are well managed by their general practitioner, with only 15–30 per cent of people being referred on to a specialist in the UK. The main reasons for referring a patient to a specialist are that the patient is unsatisfied (56 per cent) and/or the GP was uncertain of a diagnosis (35 per cent).

Tests a doctor may carry out in diagnosing IBS

It is very common for a doctor to take a blood sample. This is usually checked for:

- Blood count to check for anaemia.
- Erythrocyte sedimentation rate (ESR). This can indicate whether inflammation or tissue damage is present.

Sometimes a stool sample can be tested for an intestinal parasite or hidden (occult) blood in the stool, but most doctors do not do this unless there is good reason to do so. Other possible tests include sigmoidoscopy, colonoscopy and barium enemas; but these are really not necessary unless you and your doctor are concerned about the presence of other disorders.

Dr K. Heaton, a recognised expert on IBS, believes that 'often, no tests are needed. If the history is classical and the patient recognises a relation to stress or dietary change, it is meddlesome to do any tests. To do them could even be counterproductive, raising doubts in the patient's mind about the diagnosis and creating anxiety that can take a long time to allay' (Heaton and Thompson, 1999).

Summary

- We are not sure what causes IBS.
- Many people claim to have food intolerances and allergies but these are hard to prove and don't seem to be the cause of IBS.
- There are motility disturbances in the gut but these have not been shown to be the cause of IBS either.
- It may be that the fault lies in the nervous control of the intestine (enteric nervous system (ENS)) but further research is needed.

- IBS sufferers have been found to be more sensitive in the gut area than people without IBS and this sensitivity can set off a reaction that causes many of the IBS symptoms.
- Inflammation caused through gastroenteritis or ulcerative colitis can trigger IBS.
- Emotions such as anxiety and anger can inflame the symptoms of IBS but are not the sole cause and may be overestimated.
- IBS is not a psychiatric disorder and just because there is no identifiable abnormality found in IBS it does not mean that the symptoms are in a person's head.
- What people learn from their parents may influence the way they then deal with IBS.
- Rather than attributing the onset of IBS to one specific cause, it is more sensible to see IBS as being caused by many factors combining together.
- IBS can have a great effect on work, social and personal aspects of life.
- If you think you have IBS you should visit a doctor.

Diet

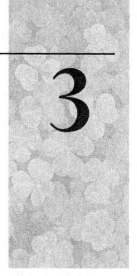

3

This chapter explores various lay theories relating to diet and IBS and includes IBS sufferers' experiences. At the end of the chapter we discuss the latest research.

A trawl through various Internet sites on the subject of IBS and diet produces some startling revelations. For instance, 'Kanga' writes from Australia that her husband has been told to try the 'BRAT' diet for his IBS. This, reveals Kanga, is Bread, Rice, Applesauce and Tea (decaf). But Kanga is immediately contradicted by 'Charlie', who insists that the BRAT diet consists of Banana, Rice, Applesauce and Toast.

The Specific Carbohydrate Diet, developed by a Dr Haas in the United States, restricts the intake of certain carbohydrates, 'thereby restoring the body's inner ecology'. This diet demands 'strict adherence' to its rules of no grains, canned and processed meats, dairy foods, canned vegetables, sugary food and starchy food, including bread, rice and pasta. On the plus side, you are allowed to eat most fresh or frozen, raw or cooked vegetables, unprocessed meat and most fruits and honey – oh, and homemade yoghurt that has been fermented for a minimum of 24 hours.

(Can we hasten to add that we do not recommend these diets. They are simply an illustration of the sorts of things you will find on the Internet.)

So is there an IBS diet?

Unfortunately, there is no one-size-fits-all IBS diet. Some people benefit from eating bran, others avoid white flour and sugar. Some people swear by virgin coconut oil for its anti-inflammatory effects, others find that restricting coffee, tea and alcohol helps.

It really is a matter of suck-it-and-see. What is important is to make sure that your diet is nourishing and well-balanced. Do not follow any diet which restricts your intake of essential nutrients. But, although there is no one diet for all people with IBS, there is dietary advice available that may help.

It is very common for people to listen to non-experts when deciding what food to restrict:

> ❝My friend told me not to eat any wheat or gluten.❞

> ❝I think I've got that thing Ginger Spice has, so I don't eat any dairy produce.❞

> ❝I know spicy food will give me the runs – I always avoid it.❞

> ❝I will not eat any food unless I can be totally sure where it came from ... I can't eat in restaurants, cafes, even cake from a friend's house is off-limits.❞

> ❝I couldn't even eat at my best friend's wedding.❞

It is also very common for people to try various restriction diets, but not reintroduce foods from previous diets, leading to an extremely restrictive and bizarre food intake:

> ❝I eat only tomatoes and plain boiled rice.❞

Another problem is that, because diets don't work, or are very difficult to maintain, people seek more and more advice and are told many different things.

Is there anything I can do to help myself?

Some people with IBS find that eating a large meal may result in severe abdominal pain or an urgent desire to go to the toilet. Eating several smaller meals during the day, rather than three large ones, may help to reduce symptoms:

> ❝I make sure I eat every two hours – I always carry around some fruit, so I do not miss a snack.❞

The most difficult foods for the body to digest are fats and animal products, so many people find it helpful to keep their meals low in fat and increase the carbohydrate content, adding more bread, pasta, rice, fruit, vegetables and cereals.

Caffeine, alcohol and citric acid are also 'no-nos' cited by many with IBS. Many juice drinks, some carbonated drinks and tomato products, as well as some packaged potato products contain citric acid. Citrus foods, especially those that are not fresh, are also avoided by some people.

Often people with IBS may link specific foods and drinks to their symptoms. These are very often idiosyncratic and associations are frequently made after just one bad experience:

> **"**I got the runs after drinking Ribena, so I avoid it totally now.**"**

This can cause moderate to severe limitations on a person's life. It is important to be aware that, just because something has caused increased symptoms, this may not happen again.

NHS Direct Online, in its self-help guide to IBS, offers the following dietary advice:

- Go for a high-fibre diet containing whole grain bread, rice and pasta.
- Eating plenty of fresh fruit can produce a remarkable long-term improvement in symptoms.
- Dairy products are often the bad guys. Try cutting out cheese, milk, chocolate, butter and cream from the diet for a few weeks to see if there is any improvement.
- Red meat, not just beef, can often seriously upset the bowel of people who are prone to IBS.
- Use herbs that are known to ease the symptoms of IBS, for example, peppermint.
- Nicotine also makes IBS much worse, so try to cut down or stop smoking altogether.
- Tea contains as much caffeine as coffee and both can cause diarrhoea in people who are prone to IBS. Coffee also contains an unknown substance that causes bowel cramps.

Food intolerance and food allergy – what are they, and is there an overlap with IBS?

Food intolerance is the general term used to describe a range of adverse responses to a specific food or food ingredient which can occur whether or not the person realises they have eaten the food. This general term includes allergic reactions that, by definition, involve the immune system (such as peanut allergy), adverse reactions resulting from enzyme deficiencies (such as lactose intolerance), pharmacological reactions (such as caffeine sensitivity) and other non-defined responses.

Food intolerance does not include food poisoning from bacteria and viruses, moulds, chemicals and toxins in food, nor food aversion (dislike and subsequent avoidance of various foods).

IBS is *not* a food allergy, but some people with IBS do discover that they are intolerant of or sensitive to particular foods. An allergy causes a very specific immunological reaction in the body that can be observed and can be diagnosed by various tests.

Food intolerance does not cause this type of reaction and cannot be tested for in the same way. This lack of a specific immune reaction and inability to test 'scientifically' has led some doctors to deny the existence of food intolerance. But, if the body cannot tolerate a certain food or foods, there is the possibility of experiencing a reaction which can range from aching joints and muscles, to wheezing, bad breath and lethargy.

What causes food intolerance?

Sometimes the cause of a food intolerance is obvious by the immediate effect that occurs on eating a particular food. In this case the treatment is simply to avoid that particular food. In most cases, however, the suspected food is more difficult to track down.

It is possible to be intolerant of:

- *complete foods*, such as milk, soya, apple, egg, pork, wheat, mushroom, chicken or lettuce; or of
- *naturally occurring chemicals*, such as salicylate in many herbs, fruit and vegetables, amines in cooked foods, purines in processed food, solanine in vegetables, tyramine in aged meat, cheeses or wines, and naturally occurring monosodium glutamate (MSG); or of
- *added ingredients*, such as preservatives, colourings, flavour or antioxidants; or of
- one of the ingredients in *processed foods*, such as wheat, preservatives, yeast or bleaching agents in bread.

Some particular offenders include:

- Sorbitol (a sugar substitute).
- Fructose (found in fruit juice and dried fruit).
- Lactose (found in milk).
- Wheat bran.

Lactose intolerance is a common condition that is the result of the body's inability to digest lactose, or milk sugar. Symptoms can include wind, bloating and, sometimes, pain. If lactose intolerance is suspected, avoidance of milk and milk products (cheese, butter, ice cream) should reduce symptoms. When milk products are reduced, however, care must be taken that enough calcium is added to the diet, either through foods high in calcium or through a calcium supplement. Yoghurt contains calcium and is, by and large, better tolerated than other milk products.

Many people with IBS say that food can bring on their symptoms. According to Nick Read, Professor of Integrated Medicine at the University of Sheffield, there is the possibility that the gut, in IBS, can be so sensitive that anything that goes into it or through it can give rise to gut feelings and cause gut reactions. But it is not yet possible to say for sure that this is the case.

> Many people worry about having food intolerances and allergies and claim that they suffer from them, even when they do not. People often say, 'I am allergic to bread', or 'I have an intolerance of pasta', but what they mean is that they had increased symptoms of IBS and associated it to the sandwich they had for lunch. They cut out the bread and the symptoms subsided – they then believed that they must have an allergy.

Food intolerances and allergies are much rarer than we think. In a recent study, only one in four of people claiming to have a food intolerance actually had one. But can something trigger intolerance to a certain food? Many reasons have been put forward to suggest why some people might have an intolerance to some foods. Perhaps they lack a particular enzyme, or maybe the intolerance is inherited, or the result of an impaired immune system, stress, environmental pollution or lack of adequate nutrition. Professor Read suggests that, in some people, food intolerance is triggered by a specific event that may be associated with food. IBS can be provoked by an attack of food poisoning, but not everyone who has food poisoning develops long-term symptoms of IBS (Dancey and Backhouse, 1997).

Most people recover without any long-term effects but, in about 30 per cent of people, the symptoms of food poisoning can go on for months or years after the original infection has cleared up. This is much more likely to occur if the original attack of food poisoning is associated with emotional upset. In these cases, the experience of food intolerance can set up psychological associations that can prove very resistant to treatment.

In other patients, the connection between emotion, food and gut symptoms may have been established early in childhood. Children can seem to go off certain foods with alarming regularity. If, however, they are made to eat up 'all those lovely carrots', they may get so upset they are sick, and never eat carrots again – an aversive association is set up between the food, the emotion and the symptom that is activated whenever the same food is presented in the future.

Box 7. Common foods that may trigger food intolerance.

- Alcohol.
- Artificial sweeteners.
- Artificial fat.
- Carbonated drinks.
- Coffee (even decaffeinated).
- Dairy.
- Egg yolks.
- Fried foods.
- Oils.
- Poultry skin and dark meat.
- Red meat.
- Chocolate.

Keeping a food diary may help with identifying the foods that cause problems. However, the British Nutrition Foundation (BNF) recommends that any food intolerance should be investigated with the help of a nutritionist or doctor. Sensitivities may be overlooked without the help of a trained professional. The BNF also warns that eliminating key foods, and, consequently, unbalancing the diet, frequently does more harm than good.

Eminent gastroenterologist John Hunter, who has carried out a great deal of work investigating food intolerances, believes it is only safe to tackle food intolerance in IBS under the supervision of a qualified specialist. A growing number of sufferers are consulting unqualified practitioners and, as a result, a number of people with IBS have been arriving at hospital outpatient departments sick and malnourished, following diets which are nutritionally inadequate.

Does eating fibre help with IBS?

One of the most common pieces of advice given to people with IBS is the exhortation to 'Eat More Fibre!' But there are, in fact, two types of fibre – soluble fibre, which can be dissolved in water, and insoluble fibre, which does not dissolve.

Insoluble fibre is 'rough', passing intact through the intestinal tract, increasing the frequency, water content and looseness of bowel movements. It can trigger painful attacks in IBS sufferers, with severe cramps that can result in diarrhoea or constipation.

By contrast, soluble fibre is smooth and soothing to the digestive tract. It absorbs excess water in the colon, forming a 'gel' which pushes through impacted faecal matter, stabilising and regulating intestinal contractions.

Foods that are naturally high in soluble fibre include oatmeal, pasta, rice, potatoes, soy, barley and oat bran. Nuts, beans and lentils are also good sources of soluble fibre but need to be treated with a degree of caution, as nuts are high in fats and both beans and lentils contain some insoluble fibre.

Insoluble fibre, although absolutely crucial for good health, can be a powerful IBS trigger. It needs to be incorporated into the diet, but not eaten alone or on an empty stomach. To incorporate raw fruit and vegetables (important for a healthy diet but high in insoluble fibre) into the diet, it might be an idea to peel and eat them in small quantities, or finely chop them and add them to high soluble fibre foods, such as rice or pasta-based dishes.

Whole wheat and bran are extremely high in insoluble fibre and foods such as whole wheat breads and cereals need to be eaten with care. But this does not mean they should not be eaten. The more whole grains that are eaten the better – overall good health is dependent on insoluble fibre. But they need to be eaten carefully – not on an empty stomach, or in large quantities or without soluble fibre foods.

Should I just stop eating certain things altogether?

CASE STUDY CASE STUDY CASE STUDY CASE STUDY

'Kath' noticed that, for several years, eating garlic gave her wind. But, the other night, she ate a quiche with fresh garlic in it and got terrible pains soon afterwards. She describes the pain as 'severe cramps or contractions in my lower bowels . . . I had to lie down and writhe on the floor'. Eventually the pain went away . . . but she had wind, for several hours, every 30 seconds, smelling like garlic. 'I think I will do a test and eat it alone without other foods,' she suggests. 'Maybe I will do several trials, just so the doctor will take me seriously . . . .'

Each item of food that is eaten is incredibly complex. Fresh fruit and vegetables, for instance, contain over 500 000 different natural compounds that produce flavour, texture, appearance and nutrient content. Over the years we have identified which foods are 'safe' to eat – that is, those which will not lead to poisoning. But, even though we may not die from eating a particular food, we can still have a sensitivity to one.

Even if the same food has been eaten every day for years, it will not be known if it is causing a problem. The only way to know that there is a food intolerance/food sensitivity problem is to eliminate suspect foods from the diet and then test them. This is the only way of knowing for sure that a particular food is a problem.

How can I carry out this test?

Trying to remember what was eaten, when and what the feeling was at the time it was eaten is never easy. Keeping a *food diary*, a detailed record of food eaten and tested and feelings/health during that time, may be the best way of testing whether there is an intolerance to certain foods.

But, to be serious about food testing, it is necessary to keep a detailed record of *everything* that is eaten. A food diary is the record of the changes that take place.

To make a food diary, buy a notebook and mark out the pages so that the foods (all the ingredients) eaten can be written down on one side and the feelings at the time can be recorded opposite. Allocate a page to each day. The diary is the evidence – keep it legible so that, if it needs to be shown to a doctor, they can read it.

Discovering what foods will help IBS can be a challenge. At times it will be difficult to follow the diet, especially if other people are not sensitive to an individual's needs. It may be hard for each individual and the people around them

---

Box 8. Foods related to intolerance.

- Dairy products (excluding live yoghurt).
- Wheat products – possible wheat sensitivity and insoluble fibre.
- Fibre-enriched foods – high content of insoluble fibre.
- Skins and pips – tomatoes, berries, figs, raisins, nuts and seeds, whole peas.
- Intestinal irritants – citrus fruits, tomatoes, chilli and spicy foods, caffeine, carbonated drinks.
- Smoked and processed foods – sensitivity to food additives.
- Wind-creating foods – lentils (whole), beans, onions, garlic, cabbage-family vegetables.
- Alcohol.

to accept. But it may be even worse to deal with an IBS attack caused by trigger foods or heavy meals.

Lactose intolerance

Lactose intolerance is the inability to digest significant amounts of lactose, the main sugar in milk. A shortage of the enzyme lactase prevents milk sugar from being broken down into simpler forms that can be easily absorbed by the bloodstream. When milk sugar is not broken down in the small intestine, it is passed to the large intestine, where it is fermented by bacteria. This fermentation is what can produce some of the symptoms of IBS. The symptoms of lactose intolerance – abdominal discomfort, bloating, wind, diarrhoea, nausea, very bad breath – can begin from 30 minutes to 2 hours after ingestion and can last for up to 3 days. The majority of people with lactose intolerance can still tolerate moderate amounts of dairy produce, such as a small glass of milk, especially if consumed as part of a meal. Hard cheese contains little lactose and so is well tolerated. For people who are very sensitive, lactose-reduced milks are now available.

Fructose intolerance

Fructose, a natural sugar present mostly in fruit, is often used to replace cane sugar. However, fructose intolerance, characterised by diarrhoea, abdominal pains and bloating, can occur after eating fructose-rich foods such as fruit, fruit juices or pure fructose. With a fructose intolerance, IBS symptoms can be aggravated.

Dietary fat

Intestinal contractions may be exaggerated in people with IBS after eating a high-fat meal such as deep-fried foods, foods with fatty meats and creamy sauces. Too much fatty food can lead to diarrhoea, so the fat content of a diet should be within normal healthy recommendations.

Sorbitol

Sorbitol, an artificial sweetener used in some sugar-free chewing gums and mints, can cause diarrhoea if too much is eaten.

Wheat/wheat bran

Wheat bran is highly controversial in the treatment of IBS. It has been found that IBS symptoms, such as diarrhoea, constipation and abdominal pain, can be exacerbated with the inclusion of wheat bran in the diet and the possibility of wheat bran causing or aggravating inflammation is being investigated. Some sufferers of IBS also seem to have fewer symptoms when they reduce their intake of wheat-based products.

Gluten intolerance

Gluten is a protein found in wheat, rye, oats and barley. According to research done in the United States in the past 10–15 years, gluten could possibly be at the root of a number of health problems, most notably coeliac disease, but including IBS. Gluten-sensitive people lack an enzyme—glutaminase – which digests the protein gluten. A strict gluten-free diet – a change from wheat-based products to corn-based items – must be followed. It is a very healthy diet as it avoids a lot of processed foods and uses a great deal of fresh foods.

Caffeine intolerance

Caffeine is so readily available in coffee, tea and chocolate that we have come to accept it as harmless, but even a relatively moderate amount, for instance two to three cups a day, can cause problems. Coffee is a bowel stimulant and many people rely on a morning cup of coffee to help them go to the toilet. If, however, diarrhoea is a symptom of IBS and a good deal of coffee is consumed, it will be necessary to cut it down or to stop completely. Even decaffeinated coffee can affect the gut. When reducing intake of caffeine-rich products, do so over a week or two, otherwise unpleasant caffeine-withdrawal symptoms, such as severe headaches, may result.

Amines

Amines are naturally occurring chemicals in certain foods which are cumulative in the body. Over a period of time these can build up in the system, causing reactions that may mimic allergies. A sensitivity to amines can often be misinterpreted as an intolerance specific to one type of food. For example, if toast doesn't agree with the system, it is easy to think that wheat is the problem; if a grilled steak causes an upset stomach then it is possible to believe there is a problem with beef when, in fact, the problem could be amines.

What else might be causing problems?

Smoking

Smoking a cigarette increases the contraction of the colon muscles in those with IBS.

> ❝I always use a fag to get my bowels open, it's the only thing that works.❞

Alcohol

Alcohol can sometimes cause diarrhoea, although generally this mostly happens to heavy drinkers. Some alcoholic drinks may aggravate IBS because of a sensitivity to yeast. This is possible with beer, especially those 'yeasty' real ales. But it is the amount that is an important factor. Don't avoid all alcohol if you like a drink.

Candida

Candida albicans is a yeast which lives in our intestines and other areas of the body, such as the skin. It is kept in check by our immune system and by 'friendly' bacteria which live with it. However, the candida can grow and get out of control when the hormonal balance of the body is disturbed, such as when following antibiotic therapy. It can spread and put down roots into the walls of the intestines. The damage to the intestinal walls allows toxins to enter the bloodstream. Symptoms in the intestines may include diarrhoea or constipation, bloatedness, flatulence and an itchy anus.

Once through to the rest of the body, candida can live anywhere there are mucous membranes – it particularly likes the vagina, lungs and the sinuses, providing food for bacteria and viruses. It has an ability to disrupt the endocrine system, causing symptoms such as weight gain or weight loss, menstrual irregularities, joint pains and chronic tiredness. Testing usually reveals vitamin, mineral and enzyme deficiencies and low blood sugar.

Both males and females suffer from candida but, overwhelmingly, it is a female condition. It would appear that at least 60 per cent of sufferers are women, 20 per cent are men and 20 per cent are boys and girls. It is regularly cited that hormonal pills (contraceptive pill or hormone replacement therapy including 'natural' progesterone cream) are the major factors in women developing candida.

Other causes of candida might include:

- Other corticosteroids (hydrocortisone, beconase, etc.).
- Hormonal changes (puberty, sexual maturity, pregnancy, sterilisation, menopause).
- Broad-spectrum antibiotics.
- Dental mercury amalgam poisoning.
- Chemical poisoning at home or work.
- Stress (usually as a contributory factor).

How can I tell whether I might have candida overgrowth?

It is not the only condition that produces these symptoms. However, according to the National Candida Society, if you have more than one *main* symptom and several of the *minor* symptoms and can link these symptoms to at least of one the *causes* in the checklist (see Box 9), then candida *may* be involved in your illness.

| Box 9. | National Candida Society: checklist. |

Main symptoms checklist (more than one).

- Have you had thrush (oral or vaginal) more than once?
- Have you had recurrent cystitis or other vaginal infections (not thrush)?
- Do you have a history of endometriosis?
- Have you had athlete's foot or fungal infections of the nails or skin?
- Are you severely affected by exposure to chemical fumes, perfumes, tobacco smoke, etc? Or are your symptoms worse after taking yeasty or sugary foods or drinks?
- Do you suffer from a variety of food allergies?
- Do you suffer from abdominal bloating, diarrhoea or constipation?
- Do you suffer from premenstrual syndrome?
- Do you suffer from depression, fatigue, lethargy or poor memory?
- Do you have food cravings?
- Do you have muscular aches, tingling, numbness or burning?
- Do you suffer from unaccountable aches and/or swelling in joints?
- Do you have erratic vision or spots before the eyes?
- Do you suffer from impotence or lack of sexual desire?

Minor symptoms checklist (several).

- Symptoms usually worse on damp days.
- Persistent drowsiness/tired all the time.
- Lack of coordination.
- Headaches/migraines.
- Mood swings.
- Loss of balance.
- Rashes.
- Mucus in stools.

- Belching and/or flatulence.

- Bad breath.

- Dry mouth or throat.

- Nasal itch and/or congestion.

- Nervous irritability.

- Tightness in chest.

- Ear sensitivity or fluid in ear.

- Heartburn and indigestion.

Causes checklist (at least one).

- Have you ever had an infection treated by antibiotics for eight weeks or more, or had antibiotics for short periods four or more times in a year?

- Have you ever taken a course of antibiotics for the treatment of acne for a month or more continuously?

- Have you ever had a course of steroid treatment, such as prednisone or cortisone?

- Have you ever taken the contraceptive pill for a year or more?

- Have you ever been treated with immuno-suppressant drugs?

- Have you had multiple pregnancies?

Food intake and IBS – what are the research facts?

There may be many nutritional influences that trigger and maintain an irritable bowel, but there is still plenty of research to do in this area. Often, people with IBS report reactions to many foods and it is hard to establish a clear link between the food and the symptoms of IBS. Below is a synopsis of research in this area.

Allergic reactions

The role of allergic food reactions in IBS has been disputed. However, there is research which indicates that there is definitely an influence.

In a study of 375 adult patients with digestive problems, it was found that 32 per cent complained of adverse reactions to food as a cause of their abdominal problems. In 14.4 per cent, the diagnosis of intestinal food allergy could be confirmed by laboratory testing. This suggests that allergic reactions to food may be a causative factor in IBS (Bischoff *et al.*, 1996).

Elimination diets

Researchers have also looked at elimination diets as a treatment of IBS. The results of one study showed that symptoms related to IBS (diarrhoea-type) improved in 60 per cent of patients treated with the elimination diet (Stefanini *et al.*, 1995). In a second study, 200 patients (156 women) with IBS underwent a 3-week elimination diet. Of the 189 who completed the study, 91 (48.2 per cent) showed symptomatic improvement (Nanda *et al.*, 1989).

Dairy products

Dairy products are often identified as an important factor contributing to an irritable bowel. The effect of a lactose-free diet was studied on 230 patients with IBS. Dairy intake problems were seen in 157 patients (68.2 per cent). There was a significant improvement in 48 (43.6 per cent) of the 100 patients who complied with the diet. In 43 patients the symptoms were somewhat reduced and in 17 they remained unchanged. Those patients who did not comply with the diet did not show any improvement in symptoms (Vernia *et al.*, 1995).

Refined sugar

Increasing consumption of refined sugar has been implicated in many digestive disorders. A research study compared the effects of a diet containing 165 grams of refined sugar per day, with a diet of only 60 grams per day. In the high-sugar diet, mouth-to-anus time was significantly prolonged, indicating a tendency to produce constipation. Breath hydrogen tests showed significantly enhanced hydrogen production on the high-sugar diet. High hydrogen production is an indication of malabsorption (Kruis *et al.*, 1991).

Fructose and sorbitol

Another study looked at the influence of fructose, sorbitol and a fructose–sorbitol combination. Ingestion of fructose caused marked abdominal distress in patients. Sorbitol had the same effect. Ingestion of sucrose in these patients gave less pronounced symptoms of abdominal distress. Mixtures of fructose and of sorbitol also caused significantly increased abdominal distress. This study showed that pronounced gastrointestinal distress may be provoked by malabsorption of small amounts of fructose, sorbitol and fructose–sorbitol mixtures in patients with functional bowel disease (Rumessen and Gudmand-Hoyer, 1988).

Fats

Fat acts as a major dietary stimulant for the colon. Patients with IBS react excessively to a fatty meal, increasing the frequency of watery stool. This relationship was more pronounced in patients who had diarrhoea as a major symptom. On the other hand, patients who had constipation as a major complaint were found to be less reactive to a fatty meal (Kellow *et al.*, 1988).

Summary

- If you do feel you have intolerance to certain foods, be as systematic as possible about testing it out. Just because something makes your symptoms worse once does not mean it is related to your IBS.

- IBS is not a food allergy.

- There are many varied diets that claim to help IBS. Most are unlikely to provide a miracle cure.

- There is no one diet for all people with IBS.

- It is vital our diet is nourishing and well-balanced. Do not follow any diet which is not.

- A constant, regular, well-balanced diet may help reduce some of the IBS symptoms.

- Make sure that any dietary advice you take is given by a medically recognised health professional.

- Do not become obsessed with the role of diet. Constantly fluctuating your diet will lead to fluctuating pain and discomfort.

Medical treatments

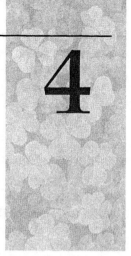

In this chapter we examine the range of medical treatments that can be called upon to control symptoms in IBS.

'Sue' is 33 years old and, according to her message on an IBS bulletin board, she has had severe IBS for around five years. 'It is ruining my life,' she says. 'Some days I could just sit back and cry because I can't take not feeling well any more.' She has also had 'so many tests that I could probably administer them myself'. But have the doctors she has seen been helpful? 'No!', she exclaims. 'One actually told me that some doors squeak and others don't. I just happen to have a squeaky door.'

Another response on the same bulletin board tells of doctors 'treating me like a hypochondriac'. Yet another writes: 'Doctors don't give me much help. They just want to poke and pry . . . and I'm tired of it.'

Members of the medical profession are confronted with patients with the troublesome and persistent symptoms of IBS on a very regular basis and medical science has long been baffled by the problem.

As highlighted in Chapter 1, it has been estimated that as many as one-third of people in Britain have occasional symptoms of IBS and between 10 and 20 per cent have symptoms bad enough to require medical attention. This is an extremely high figure for a disorder for which no organic cause can be found. IBS costs the NHS many millions of pounds each year and is responsible for much human distress.

The fact that IBS has a multitude of possible causes and that its manifestation can vary from individual to individual, added to the further complication that it does not involve any obvious physical disease, means that the best most doctors can offer is a reassurance that the condition is not life-threatening and prescriptions for medications which will relieve some of the symptoms.

Although there is no one, single treatment for IBS which works for all of the people, all of the time, there is a range of different treatments which work well for many people at various times.

> As long ago as 1988, Klein declared that 'not a single study has been published that provides compelling evidence that any therapeutic agent is efficacious in the global treatment of IBS' (Klein, 1988). Little has changed since this oft-quoted critique of IBS clinical trials was made.

However, although the cause of IBS is not yet fully understood, recent research has revealed that the bowel in IBS sufferers is likely to be more sensitive than usual and this sensitivity sets off a reaction which causes the symptoms. Michael Gershon, a senior American anatomist and cell biologist, believes nerve transmissions between the brain and the nerves lining the walls of the intestines mean that the mind and the gut 'talk' to one another. The brain sends signals to the digestive system and influences activity there. And, he says, the reverse is true: any distress felt in the bowels can also cause mental distress (Gershon, 1998).

As already mentioned in Chapter 2 (p. 20), in a study at the University College of Los Angeles, IBS patients were tested by inflating balloons in their intestines and pain sensitivity levels were measured, together with the amount of tension in the muscles of the intestines before and after the balloon treatment. There were altered responses by both the brain and the gut to balloon inflation in the intestines. The brain responses were measured using an imaging technique called positron emission tomography (PET) and, in IBS patients, the brain responded to the stresses and stimuli in the gut differently than in healthy individuals, confirming, stated the researchers, that there is a definite brain/gut connection with IBS (Moore, no date).

In another study at the University of Washington in Seattle, researchers discovered that physiological distress was a key factor in at least 40 per cent of women with IBS who were tested (Moore, no date).

To reiterate and reinforce earlier explanations, IBS is a benign disorder of the way in which the bowel functions. For this reason, it is often referred to as a 'functional bowel disorder'. This means that, so far as is currently known, the condition, while displaying an abnormality of the function of the bowel, does not arise from any structural change in it or from any organic disease process. This does not mean that it is imaginary. However, there is no accurate test for IBS. It is diagnosed when a doctor has excluded other possible causes for the symptoms.

Box 10.

Guidelines for the diagnosis have been proposed by the NHS. They suggest that the affected person should, for at least 12 weeks in the last 12 months, have suffered abdominal discomfort or pain for which no organic cause is found. The 12 weeks need not be continuous but may be a total. The person should also show two of the following three features:

- Pain is relieved by defecation (passing a motion).
- Pain is associated with a change in the frequency of bowel movement, either an increase or a decrease.
- There is a change in the form of the stool – it is watery, loose or pellet-like.

IBS provides specialists in bowel disorders – gastroenterologists – with over 60 per cent of their patients. This does not mean that IBS represents 60 per cent of all bowel disorders – only of the ones referred to a specialist. Gastroenterologists see many of these cases because of the high proportion referred to them by GPs.

Although IBS may produce unpleasant and often embarrassing symptoms, it does not lead to serious complications. It is important to know and understand this. An explanation of the disorder and how symptoms are produced helps to relieve anxiety and means symptoms may be easier to cope with. If attacks are infrequent, or mild, this insight may be enough.

Box 11.

It has been observed that there are various levels of treating IBS. At the **first level**, most people do not consult a GP. They manage with their symptoms and get on with their lives. It has been estimated that the majority of people with IBS are never formally diagnosed. Many people believe that a doctor cannot do much for the condition, so they simply get on with things.

At the **second level**, people go to their GP when their symptoms are particularly troublesome or persistent, especially if they have considerable pain, or if they think they may have something more serious ('Dad had bowel cancer'). Often reassurance that they do not have anything serious is enough.

If this does not work, at the **third level**, some sort of medication is the usual treatment.

Finally, at the **fourth level**, a referral to a specialist – gastroenterologist – may be the next step. It depends on how anxious the doctor and the patient are.

Reassurance that more serious or progressive disorders are not present is certainly important. Knowledge of what provokes an attack may help with the more effective control of symptoms, and attacks may be prevented, or at least coped with more easily.

Medication is not a first choice for treatment of IBS. The guts of people with IBS are often as sensitive to medications as they can be to food. Besides, if a drug really worked in IBS, it would presumably be used everywhere. There is much variety and inconsistency in the drugs approved by the regulatory bodies of different countries and many people prefer, and are able, to control their symptoms with home treatment. The goal of drug treatment is to relieve symptoms enough to prevent them interfering with daily activities, because it may not be possible to eliminate symptoms altogether.

Medications may be useful to control individual *symptoms* of IBS. But, if used at all, drugs should be employed for short periods and should be closely monitored for effectiveness and side effects. Medication may be prescribed to treat moderate to severe pain, diarrhoea, or constipation that does not respond to home treatment. Antidepressant medications may improve IBS symptoms, even in people who do not have depression. Anxiety medications may help people whose anxiety contributes to their IBS symptoms. In most cases, the choice of medication is based on a person's most troublesome symptom. No single medication has been shown to be effective in relieving IBS over the long term and GPs have their own preferences about what they prescribe.

At a recent conference in the United States on functional gastrointestinal disorders, Michel Delvaux, from University Hospital Rangueil in Toulouse, France, noted that there were considerable differences between medication use for IBS in North America (primarily antispasmodics, anti-diarrhoeals and antidepressants) and in Europe (a wider variety of classes of smooth muscle relaxants and fewer antidepressants) (Delvaux, 2001).

Fibre may often be the first-line treatment offered by many doctors. But this is normally in the form of bran supplements, which can make matters worse for IBS sufferers. Bran can be useful in easing constipation – it leads to a bulkier stool which allows the bowel to push it through more quickly.

But only now is it being recognised that bran is, of course, wheat bran, and wheat may be one of the foods many IBS sufferers are intolerant of. Wheat bran is also a rather coarse product and can cause further irritation to an already sensitive bowel lining.

In contrast to natural wheat bran, manufactured fibre supplements made from plant extracts have been found to be beneficial to many people. These are slower than wheat bran to show an effect and may be better tolerated.

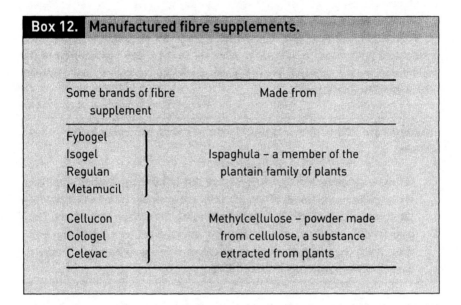

| Box 12. | Manufactured fibre supplements. |

Some brands of fibre supplement	Made from
Fybogel Isogel Regulan Metamucil	Ispaghula – a member of the plantain family of plants
Cellucon Cologel Celevac	Methylcellulose – powder made from cellulose, a substance extracted from plants

The placebo effect

There is a profound placebo response to any IBS treatment and, as scientists from the University of British Columbia in Canada have revealed, the placebo effect is not all in the mind. The UBC scientists have published results of a study which yielded evidence that a placebo could provide measurable effects in the brain for the treatment of Parkinson's disease (Highfield, 2001).

The researchers used a brain scanner to show that a placebo produced the same boost in the brain's dopamine levels as active drugs to treat Parkinson's, the neurodegenerative disorder which causes the destruction of brain cells that produce the messenger chemical dopamine.

Placebos – sometimes called dummy pills or sugar pills – are treatments that have no pharmacological properties. The placebo effect is the measurable, observable or felt improvement in health not attributable to the treatment. Patients who take a placebo should not improve, yet a substantial number do. A wealth of studies have backed up the idea that placebos – medically useless pills, potions and tonics – can often help depression, treat ulcers and relieve pain, just as well as conventional treatments. Big pills work better than small pills and coloured pills work better than white pills. Some researchers believe that the effects of many alternative therapies can also be explained by the placebo effect.

The word 'placebo', which means 'I will please' in Latin, came to mean a medicine given 'more to please than to benefit the patient' by the early nineteenth century.

Placebo effects have been seen to result simply from contact with doctors or other healthcare providers. Sometimes a diagnosis or simple attention from a respected professional is enough to alleviate anxiety. The expectations of the patient can have a powerful impact, particularly for complaints and disorders which involve chronic pain.

According to Walter Brown, a psychiatrist at Brown University in the United States:

'There is certainly data that suggest that just being in the healing situation accomplishes something. When placebos are given for pain management, the course of pain relief follows what you would get with an active drug. The peak relief comes about an hour after it is administered, as it does with a real drug. If placebo analgesia was the equivalent of giving nothing, you'd expect a more random pattern' (Talbot, 2001).

W. Grant Thompson (1989), Emeritus Professor of Medicine at the University of Ottawa, Canada, believes that 'clinical trials have failed to prove that any (drug) therapy is more beneficial overall than a placebo'.

A person's beliefs and hopes about a treatment, combined with their suggestibility, may have a significant biochemical effect – a person's hopeful attitudes and beliefs may be very important to their physical well-being and recovery from illness or injury.

So what is the explanation for the placebo effect? Some people think it is the *process* of administering the placebo – the touching, the caring, the attention and other interpersonal communication, along with the hopefulness and encouragement given by the healthcare provider. These affect the mood of the patient, which, in turn, triggers physical changes such as the release of endorphins. The process reduces stress by providing hope, or by reducing uncertainty about what treatment to take, or about what the outcome will be. The reduction in stress prevents further harmful physical changes from occurring, or slows them down.

Drugs for abdominal pain

Pain is often the dominant symptom of IBS and, along with bloating, is the symptom least amenable to drug treatment.

The pain of IBS had been thought to be related to spasm of the colonic muscle – although this notion is now discredited among many physicians – and the traditional approach has been to reduce gut spasm by prescribing antispasmodics, which vary from direct smooth muscle relaxants or preparations of peppermint oil, to a range of complex and powerful drugs known as anticholinergics.

Anticholinergic drugs have the potential to reduce abdominal pain and may be helpful when pain predictably follows a meal. However, their side effects can include constipation, nausea, vomiting, impaired vision, difficulty urinating, a dry mouth and insomnia and their efficacy in improving IBS symptoms has not yet been proved definitively.

Peppermint oil relaxes the intestine by preventing calcium entry into intestinal smooth muscle cells. Because calcium triggers the cascade of events leading to muscle contraction, the inhibition of calcium in the cells causes intestinal smooth muscle relaxation. However, more studies need to be undertaken to fully understand the role of peppermint oil in IBS treatment.

Recent studies have suggested that five drugs – cimetropium bromide, pina verium bromide, trimebutine, octilinium bromide and mebeverine, all direct smooth muscle relaxants – significantly improve IBS sufferers' overall well-being, pain and abdominal distension. Side effects appear to be rare. However, only mebeverine has a product licence in the UK.

In people whose pain is constant, and more like chronic functional abdominal pain, small doses of antidepressants may help, even in the absence of obvious depression. It is not clear why antidepressant drugs may help pain. Is it because of the drug's antidepressant properties? Or does the drug help prevent muscle spasms in the bowel wall? Or does it have a direct effect on how pain is received? At the moment, no one really has the answer.

Antidepressant drugs differ in their strength and side effects, but they do not seem to cause the same degree of dependency and withdrawal problems as tranquillisers. The drugs mostly commonly prescribed to IBS sufferers are tricyclic antidepressants (TCAs) such as desipramine, imipramine and amitryptiline. They can be useful in relieving pain in a number of chronic pain syndromes, but they can cause side effects which include dry mouth, constipation, blurred vision, drowsiness, dizziness, weight change and loss of libido.

Selective serotonin reuptake inhibitors (SSRIs), such as fluoxetine, sertraline and paroxetine, are also now commonly used to treat IBS. Tricyclic antidepressants are probably more effective for people with a loose bowel habit and SSRIs for those with constipation. SSRIs have fewer side effects than TCAs – the main ones are nausea, headaches, insomnia and sexual dysfunction.

It is important to recognise that being prescribed antidepressants as a treatment for IBS does not mean the doctor believes the disorder is caused by psychological problems – there is general agreement within the medical profession that antidepressants seem to be of unequivocal benefit to some people. A recent study concluded that antidepressants are effective in reducing the symptoms associated with IBS and with functional gastrointestinal disorders in about one-third of patients. The analgesic effects of these drugs may also occur in lower dosages than when used for the treatment of depression.

Tranquillisers, too, are prescribed for people with IBS, especially when IBS symptoms are accompanied by anxiety and panic attacks. They can be helpful if some particularly traumatic event has temporarily made symptoms very much worse. Librium (chlordiazepoxide) and Valium (diazepam) may be useful for short-term treatment. However, these drugs can cause addiction if used for any length of time; coming off them can cause a rebound effect of heightened anxiety and panic and there is a risk that they may interact with other medicines that might be taken.

In a survey of IBS sufferers carried out by Susan Backhouse and Christine Dancey, the founders of the IBS Network, most people did not feel that, on its own, antispasmodic medication helped them a great deal. According to Backhouse and Dancey, this ties in with scientific studies that have shown that combined treatment – antispasmodic, bulk filler, tranquilliser – gives better results than any one medication alone (Dancey and Backhouse, 1997).

More general painkillers, such as paracetamol, codeine phosphate and Distalgesic, have a constipating action. Painkillers are best kept, therefore, for emergencies only. Taking time to relax and rest, perhaps with a hot water bottle held close to the abdomen, can help.

Drugs for diarrhoea

Diarrhoea is the passing of increased amounts (more than 300 grams in 24 hours) of loose stools and it occurs when micro-organisms irritate the mucous membrane of the small or large intestine, resulting in an abnormally large quantity of water in the motions. The irritated gut becomes very active, contracting excessively and irregularly. Chronic diarrhoea can be a symptom of IBS. Some people are particularly troubled by sudden, unpredictable episodes of diarrhoea, and some even fear incontinence, which may make them miss social or business engagements, because of fear of embarrassment. In some cases, some people become totally reclusive and hardly ever leave the safety of their home.

Diarrhoea can usually be treated safely at home. The prophylactic use of anti-diarrhoeal drugs such as loperamide (Imodium) or diphenoxylate (Lotomil) may restore a sense of control and allow more socialization. These are quite powerful drugs and can stop the flow of the most severe diarrhoea. However, patients with severe IBS may find the treatment of diarrhoea with these drugs is accompanied by a marked increase in abdominal pain.

Too many anti-diarrhoeal tablets can lead to constipation and may lead to a see-sawing between diarrhoea and constipation – an even less pleasant prospect than having either symptom alone. The most commonly taken drug for diarrhoea is Imodium (loperamide) which can be bought over the counter. Imodium slows down the passage of waste through the system and increases absorption of water. It acts on the gut alone and is not absorbed into the system, greatly diminishing any risk of side effects. Lotomil (diphenoxylate) and codeine phosphate are absorbed and can cause side effects of drowsiness and dizziness. They may even cause dependency in some people.

Drugs for wind

Wind can be very difficult to treat. There is no definitive medical treatment for bloating, distension and flatulence, though it might be a good idea to reduce the intake of gas-forming foods, such as fruit, beans and other pulses, vegetables and cereal fibre, and to avoid bulk-forming laxatives such as Regulan.

Some of the gassiest people in the world are intolerant of lactose (milk sugar) – a reduction in milk or milk products may alleviate this symptom for some people. Excessive wind production may also be associated with carbohydrate intolerance as carbohydrates and sugars cannot be digested in the small bowel so they pass into the colon, where they are readily fermented, producing hydrogen and carbon dioxide – gas. A reduction in the amount of sugars consumed in sweets, biscuits, drinks, etc., may help. Cutting out wheat is also worth a try.

There is anecdote-based enthusiasm in North America for Beano in the treatment of wind. This enzyme alpha-galactosidase digests some carbohydrates not processed in the small intestine, and leads to the absorption of sugars without the formation of gas. Beano is not available on prescription.

Peppermint oil, cinnamon, cloves, ginger and fennel tea have also been used by some IBS sufferers with severe wind, to good effect.

Dimethylpolysiloxane (Ovol) breaks up bubbles in the secretion of the upper gut. It is available in some countries but, so far, there is little proof that this is helpful to the bloating associated with IBS.

Drugs for constipation

Constipation is caused by a hard stool which is difficult to expel, or motions which occur at intervals of several days. Symptoms of constipation include pain associated with bowel movement, a feeling of incomplete emptying of the bowel and a feeling of bloatedness in the stomach region. Chronic constipation can cause considerable distress and certainly exacerbates all the other features of IBS.

For constipation that is not helped by increasing the amount of fibre in the diet, there is a wide range of laxatives available; but these should only be used for short periods of time. They have a tendency to make the muscles of the bowel lazy, so, when the treatment stops, the problem can be worse than before.

Laxatives are divided into two main types:

- **osmotic** – osmotics, such as Duphalac (lactulose), ease constipation by drawing fluid into the bowel and so softening the stools. They should be taken with plenty of water and it is important to make sure to continue to drink a lot of fluid throughout a course of treatment. Lactulose can produce a lot of gas in IBS patients. However, a laxative effect is generally achieved in one to two days.

- **stimulant** – stimulant laxatives, such as Sennokot, Dulco-Lax and Normacol Plus, work by increasing the constricting and relaxing motion of the muscles in the bowel wall, the action known as motility, in order to push the stools through faster. The problem is that this stimulation can aggravate and even trigger the pain often felt in IBS by causing excruciating spasms of the sensitive colon. Stimulant laxatives should be used sparingly and only when osmotic laxatives have been ineffective. Stimulant laxatives take effect within hours of taking them.

There are also two types of emollient laxatives:

- **docusates** – which act by allowing a greater amount of water to enter the stool, thus softening it. They are generally well-tolerated but less effective than other laxatives.

- **mineral oil** – is a stool softener that coats the bowel and stool with a waterproof film. Moisture is then retained in the stool, making it softer and easier to pass. However, it should be used cautiously as an oral laxative by people who have difficulty swallowing, because, if inhaled into the lung, it could cause inflammation.

For constipation, many members of the IBS Network recommend eating linseed, which can be sprinkled on cereal or yoghurt or simply swallowed and works gently on the system.

Newer drugs

Some of the newer gastrointestinal drugs coming out or under investigation include agents to treat multiple symptoms, including constipation and chronic pain. Examples include the 5-HT agents – e.g. Alosetron, a 5-HT3 antagonist (which was withdrawn from the commercial market because of some serious side effects but which may return for limited use, perhaps with women with the most severe diarrhoea from IBS), Cilansetron, another 5-HT3 antagonist, and Tegaserod, a 5-HT4 receptor partial agonist. Tegaserod has been found, in studies, to relieve abdominal pain and reduce constipation in some patients. It has also proven efficacy in improving bloating and stool consistency. The M3 receptor antagonists zamifenacin and darifenacin are also under investigation as potential treatments for diarrhoea-predominant IBS. These antispasmodic selective inhibitors decrease motor activity in the gut and so may be particularly useful in IBS. The growing understanding of the neurotransmitters and receptors in disorders such as IBS is paving the way for new classes of medicines soon to be released.

Conclusion

While some people with IBS respond well to drugs, the relief from symptoms often does not last. One of the chief problems of drug treatment in IBS is the real risk of relieving one set of symptoms, only to find out that in doing so another symptom has been caused or aggravated. Unless symptoms are particularly acute and troublesome, it is probably better to avoid drugs – some of those prescribed can even be addictive if used for any length of time.

Drugs will not get to the root of the problem and they are certainly not a cure for IBS. It may be decided, therefore, to take any medication on an emergencies-only basis. However, if medications are employed long term, ask the doctor prescribing them to explain exactly how the drug works and what its potential side effects are. This may help in making a decision about its use.

Summary

- There is no one, single treatment for IBS – but a range of different treatments work for many people at different times.

- IBS is a benign disorder of the way in which the bowel functions. The condition does not arise from any structural change or organic disease in the bowel – but it is certainly NOT imaginary.

- IBS may produce unpleasant and embarrassing symptoms, but it does NOT lead to serious complications.

- Medication is not the first choice for treatment for IBS, but may be useful to control individual symptoms. Drugs for diarrhoea and constipation can help but wind and abdominal pain may be difficult to treat.

● There is a profound placebo effect for IBS – sometimes there can be improvements simply after sitting down and discussing the problem with a doctor or other health professional. The beneficial effects of some alternative therapies may also be explained by the placebo effect.

● Newer drugs currently under investigation may, in the future, be able to treat multiple symptoms of IBS, including constipation and chronic pain.

Psychological treatments

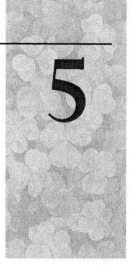

5

The aim of this chapter is to try and make sense of the role of talking treatments or psychotherapies that may be on offer for IBS. It will describe many of the main types available and evaluate the evidence for each of them.

We have seen how many people with IBS receive adequate treatment from their local doctor. This standard medical treatment should help around half of IBS sufferers. What happens to those who continue to experience severe symptoms despite the best efforts of themselves and their doctor?

There are many varied and elaborate forms of treatment for IBS on offer. Many people offering medical, psychological or alternative therapies will claim they can help, but not all of them will.

This chapter and the next one examine the psychological and alternative treatments currently available. We will describe what each consists of and have given each therapy a score out of 50 based on the following criteria; the higher the score the more we recommend the therapy.

1. Scientific research (0–20)

When we are prescribed drugs by our GP, we expect that drug to have been thoroughly tested to make sure it that it will actually help with our condition and that it is not going to cause any unforeseen side effects. Most of us assume the same things happen with psychological and alternative treatments. *They don't!* The research that is done to test out these sorts of therapies varies immensely. Some will rely on feedback from those who have had the treatment.

> 66 Well he did show me letters from others who had the treatment and they were all very complimentary to the treatment. One lady wrote 'it had changed her life', so it sounds like its worth a shot, what do you think doctor? 99

Others will claim that the treatment has been around for hundreds of years and that in itself must mean it is worthwhile. Astrology has been practised for many hundreds of years and yet, after all that time there is still absolutely no evidence that because your star is heading into the realm of Pluto 'you will have a chance meeting with an old friend today'.

For any therapy to be credible it should be willing to subject itself to be tested under scientific conditions. Many treatments have very few published studies examining their effectiveness, and many that do are vague and open to many interpretations.

We believe scientific research is the key category and therefore will give each therapy a score out of 20. To score highly in this category a therapy will have provided clear evidence that its treatment has been tested and is effective. Low scores mean that we found it difficult to find any real evidence that this therapy works for IBS.

2. Availability (0–10)

High scores mean that the treatment is either readily available on the National Health Service or easily found in most high streets. Low scores suggest that the treatment is only available in few specialised centres around the country.

3. Cost (0–10)

High scores will denote the treatment is free or fairly cheap; low scores suggest that the treatment is either expensive, over-priced or a complete rip-off.

4. Attractiveness (0–10)

Many people are moving away from traditional Western medicine and treatments and looking for something different. Treatments such as massage can be very pleasant and an enjoyable experience to undergo. To get a good score in this category the treatment should be highly acceptable, believable and attractive to the person undergoing it. Low scores denote the treatment may be difficult, uncomfortable, etc.

It seems we really can't get enough of talking therapy. Television is full of counsellors and therapists spouting forth advice on how to deal with all manner of life issues. There are almost as many of them as there are cooks and decorators. Many of these therapists also believe that they have something to offer the world of IBS. In previous chapters we have already described how many of the symptoms experienced in IBS can be triggered by stress, so it does seem to make some sense that they may be able to help. What are the different types? Do they work? Let's look at the evidence.

The overlap

We will describe three different forms of psychotherapy. Each has its own way of approaching IBS and offers different ways to beat it, but all have similarities and a degree of overlap.

All psychotherapies rely on a good relationship between the therapist and the person (or, as therapists often call them, 'client'). This does not mean that it is necessary to be best friends, but it is important to feel comfortable and respected and to have trust in the therapist's expertise. Not getting on with the therapist means a possibility of poor results from the treatment. This does not necessarily mean that the treatment does not work; it may simply be necessary to try another therapist.

It is important to be able to understand what therapists are saying; they should not be over-complicated or use medical jargon (see Chapter 7 for jargon busting). They should also have a good working knowledge of IBS and problems associated with it.

The aim of these sorts of therapies is the understanding that we have the power within us to beat IBS. The different psychological treatments use different ways to try and show us how to do this.

Hypnotherapy

What is hypnotherapy?

A hypnotist on the television is often seen as having some amazing power and control over whoever is under hypnosis, making them do weird and stupid things like eating an onion as if it were a juicy apple, all for the amusement of the baying crowd. This popular view of hypnosis is a long way from the truth and very different from the way hypnosis is used clinically.

Clinical hypnosis is a way of helping a person achieve a special state of mind. Using various relaxing techniques the therapist will help the person achieve this trance-like state of deep relaxation. The mind is then really focused and responsive to suggestions and ideas. The person having the hypnosis is almost always totally aware of what happens under hypnosis during and after the session. The treatment is usually without side effects, but the hypnotist should be aware of any ongoing psychiatric illness. This is why it is important you make sure you receive treatment not only from a qualified hypnotherapist but preferably one who has a medical or health background as well.

Gut-directed hypnotherapy

There are many types of hypnotherapy available, but gut-directed hypnotherapy has been specially designed to work with IBS. Dr Peter Whorwell and colleagues from Manchester first described the process of gut-directed hypnotherapy in 1984.

The process of gut-directed hypnosis

There is more to gut-directed hypnosis than just hypnosis. People are usually given a tutorial with a doctor all about IBS to begin with, looking at our current understanding of the syndrome, what we think is currently going on, and how they may be able to improve the symptoms.

Then the therapist teaches the person to use progressive muscular relaxation to achieve the state of hypnosis. Once a good level of hypnosis has been achieved the person is encouraged to visualise their IBS and use specific techniques to help improve it.

For a person suffering from constipation the therapist may ask the person to see their guts as a river:

> **❝**Imagine your gut is a stagnant river, its waters are murky, still and clogged, dank and dark in the dead of winter. Now imagine the river starting to flow, gently at first, through green grassy meadows on a warm summers day and streams, it starts to quicken, bubbling across the pebbles, under a bridge and into a valley. The river has widened, rolling down to the wide open sea.**❞**

And likewise if the person suffers from diarrhoea:

> **❝**Imagine your bowels as a fast-flowing river with strong currents and eddies, swirling and raging, now calm the stream down, it's slowing down and the current is weak . . . . **❞**

This can be a very effective treatment; as one hypnotherapist wrote:

> **❝**I remember using hypnosis to treat constipation in a rather sombre woman of 21. I suggested that we imagine her river as shallow and flowing merrily over pebbles in the bright sunlight. The following week, she came back with a merry little attack of diarrhoea and I had to slow the river down.**❞**

They are then asked to take home an audiotape of a session, listen to it and carry out the instructions on a daily basis. Over time they can often learn how to do it without the need for a therapist.

Treatment lasts on average 12 sessions on a weekly basis and each session takes between 30 and 40 minutes. In fact fewer than 7 sessions have been shown to be less effective. Sometimes, after the treatment is finished, people are able to get booster sessions by phone.

Does it work?

Dr Peter Whorwell's first study in 1984 (Whorwell *et al.*, 1984) demonstrated great success with 15 people with severe IBS that had not improved with previous treatments.

All the major symptoms of IBS improved with gut-directed hypnosis – pain, constipation, diarrhoea and bloating. This led to great improvements in people's general well-being and quality of life. Since that time over a dozen studies have been published agreeing that his form of hypnosis is an effective (around 70–90 per cent) and long-lasting (at least two years).

These trials have been carried out in a clear scientific manner. The treatment has been shown to be effective in groups as well as on an individual basis. Dr Whorwell writes (Whorwell *et al.*, 1987):

> **❝**All the data suggests that hypnosis is a very good treatment for severe IBS and it is tempting to speculate that milder persons might even do better.**❞**

How does it work?

No one is really sure how hypnosis really works; Dr Whorwell has written:

> **❝**the mechanism by which hypnotherapy helps these persons must remain speculative at this time but, undoubtedly, there must be a powerful psychotherapeutic component to a treatment of this type.**❞**

Where is the catch?

The good news and the bad news . . .

The good news is that gut-directed hypnotherapy is an excellent, long-lasting and well-researched treatment for severe IBS. The bad news is that it is costly to provide, time-consuming and labour-intensive for the people carrying it out. This means it can be hard to obtain. There are some people that do not seem to benefit at all, for example some people with psychiatric disorders. Also about 20 per cent of us find it difficult to be hypnotised and will not be able to achieve the state of mind needed for the techniques to work. Taking all these things into account it is unlikely that hypnotherapy will be a solution for the majority of IBS sufferers.

A word about other types of hypnotherapy

Watch out for other types of hypnotherapy.

There is not just one form of hypnotherapy. For hypnosis to be effective it should be focused on the gut (gut-directed hypnotherapy). Sometimes people's experience of hypnosis has not been specific to the gut.

Some people have used the successful results of gut-directed hypnotherapy to suggest that their form of hypnosis is also successful. This has yet to be demonstrated and it is important to be wary. An example of this is hypnosis where the hypnotist either tries to 'regress' the person to a much younger age, when a traumatic incident may have occurred, or in some cases tries to 'go back much further' to a supposed 'previous life'.

One woman, who had experienced this form of hypnotherapy, explained that the hypnotist took her back to a previous life in the Middle Ages where she was a male tax-collector. In this life she suffered from severe stomach pains and diarrhoea. The hypnotist spent several sessions curing this 'man' via hypnosis. It had little effect on the woman's IBS, which continued in much the same way. It did, however, have a great effect on her bank balance. The whole treatment promised so much, gave so little and cost a packet!

It is important you select your hypnotherapist carefully. Many people who practise hypnotherapy are not qualified to treat medical problems. Don't be taken in by the often-impressive-looking letters after someone's name. If they are not a health professional (doctor, nurse, psychologist, psychiatrist, social worker, etc.) they may not have had formal training. Ask them about this. Hypnosis by itself is not enough to help IBS, so ask the therapist if they are aware of gut-directed hypnosis.

Scientific research	16
Availability	3
Cost	7 (can be found on the NHS)
Attractiveness	8
Total score	*34*

Psychodynamic psychotherapy

What is psychodynamic psychotherapy?

Psychodynamic psychotherapy is the nearest to most people's traditional view of psychotherapy. Within the sessions, a trained psychotherapist will listen to the person talk about their problems, creating an intense personal relationship between the therapist and client (or 'patient' as they call them) so they can discuss and share their innermost fears and feelings.

The process of psychodynamic psychotherapy

The person undergoing psychotherapy will be encouraged to speak, often freely and openly. The psychotherapist will listen and, at some point in the therapy, ask for more information or ask specific questions depending on their interpretation of what is said.

The underlying theory behind this sort of therapy suggests that problems in the person's life either cause the symptoms of IBS or make them worse. The therapist believes that common problems may be related to difficulties in people's relationships, for example the loss of a parent, or the failure to form, or keep, happy and stable relationships with friends, partners or family. The creation of an intensive relationship is important because, once established, they believe that the problems in the patient's life are then 'mirrored' or recur in this relationship within the therapy sessions.

Dr Elspeth Guthrie an expert in psychodynamic psychotherapy for IBS describes an example of this (Guthrie *et al.*, 1991):

> ❝A patient may have problems in coping with authority figures, and thus develop bowel symptoms before he/she has to present a report to a supervisor. The patient may fear criticism and humiliation by the supervisor, even if in reality he/she is not overly critical. In psychotherapy, a patient with these kinds of problems will come to perceive the doctor as authoritarian, harsh and critical, even if in reality the doctor is kind and supportive.❞

The aim of this form of psychotherapy is to help the person identify these misconceptions and distortions in relationships and then learn to recognise the link between them and the IBS symptoms. Once understood, the theory suggests that this will lead to a reduction in symptoms and a better understanding by the patient of how to cope with future relationships. This in turn should lead to a lessening of IBS symptoms in the future.

Does it work?

There have been a few studies examining this kind of psychodynamic psychotherapy and they have shown that this approach can be of some benefit to some people. The trials have been fairly well conducted, although some people have criticised the measures used to demonstrate improvement. Patients seem to do better with this sort of therapy if they have associated psychiatric symptoms such as anxiety and depression and if they recognise that their symptoms are related to their stress. People who have a lot of pain associated with the IBS, or who have had IBS for over five years, seem to do less well with this approach.

This form of psychotherapy can be difficult to obtain and is time-consuming for the person involved. It is usually very hard work and can be an extremely frustrating and draining process to go through.

The problem with psychodynamic psychotherapy

> ❝I told the therapist that I had a dream about smoking. I know that smoking often helps me with constipation. In my dream I was putting a cigarette out in an ashtray. The therapist told me the dream was symbolic, the cigarette was me and the ashtray was my mother, I was pushing myself on my mother!❞

The man (above) who told me of his experience with psychodynamic psychotherapy did not return to finish off treatment; he found the whole thing fairly absurd. I have too. When I was training as a nurse I spent a week with some psychodynamic therapists at a special unit for children. At a case conference four of them were discussing a picture that a young girl had drawn of herself. It was a simple line drawing of a little girl with a semi-circle drawn from one hand under her legs and up to her other hand. They were discussing and interpreting how the line from hand to hand must have been done to protect her lower body from any outside influences, and suggested that this must mean she is afraid of some interference in that area. I thought it looked like a skipping-rope. As I was only a student nurse, I thought I must be ignorant not to realise that it was something more symbolic so I never questioned them. But the more I look back, the more I am sure it was a skipping-rope.

This example highlights many of the problems with interpretive psychotherapy; the interpretations made are based on the therapist's judgement and experience. This can be a hit-and-miss process. Often, if you disagree with the therapist, they use the fact that you disagree as more evidence that their theory is correct and claim you are only disagreeing because you do not want to face the truth.

Even though this form of therapy is fairly widespread throughout the world, the whole underlying premise of dynamic psychotherapy has yet to be demonstrated. There is no evidence that these theories or ways of encouraging change have any basis in reality. It is a huge and powerful industry, determined to keep its grip on the psychotherapy world. They demand their form of therapy is given equal footing to many others that have been shown to be more effective. Anyone wanting to become a psychodynamic therapist has to undergo and pay for their own psychotherapy; this currently accounts for over one-quarter of all people who have ever had therapy.

Scientific research	8
Availability	6
Cost	3 (cost varies but can be expensive)
Attractiveness	4
Total score	*21*

Cognitive behavioural psychotherapy (CBT)

What is cognitive behavioural psychotherapy?

Cognitive behavioural psychotherapy is a form of psychotherapy in which the therapist and client collaborate to find and learn ways to cope with problems and help people to live their life in the way they want to. A CBT therapist's aim is not to cure IBS – it is an enduring problem. This means that, even after experiencing CBT, there will still be symptoms. Treatment does not focus on the cause or onset of IBS. The focus of CBT is the behaviours, thoughts and feelings that surround the IBS. By improving these, CBT therapists believe that this will in turn reduce the physical symptoms of IBS.

CASE STUDY CASE STUDY CASE STUDY CASE STUDY

An example of how the way a person thinks act and feels can intensify and maintain IBS.

Tricia has an important meeting with her boss in the morning that causes her some anxiety. [feelings and thoughts]

She knows that these sorts of situations often cause her IBS to flare up, and cause more diarrhoea and bloating than usual.

She is further concerned that her diarrhoea will cause her to leave the meeting early and that she may inadvertently pass wind causing great embarrassment. [thought]

She decides to call in sick to work with diarrhoea. [behaviour]

She then feels guilty and depressed about the effect of her IBS on her life. [feelings and thoughts]

Tricia thinks that maybe she should give up her job if she can't manage to go to meetings. [behaviour and thoughts]

From the example we can see how the role of a person's thoughts, feelings and behaviours will affect how they respond to the symptoms. This, in turn, will affect many aspects of their daily life. If person experiences a particularly nasty bout of symptoms, this can cause them to focus on the symptoms much more (becoming hypersensitive to them) which then increases the impact and frequency of the IBS symptoms. This is referred to in CBT as symptoms focusing.

The process of CBT

CBT is structured so that it is possible to be clear about what is happening and where the treatment is going. The therapist outlines what is involved in treatment, identifying the treatment techniques and working towards these in a graded fashion. The client is expected to play an active and important part in treatment. What the person does between sessions – working on various issues – is just as important as what happens in the session. Ideally they should learn to become their own therapist.

Treatment is usually short-term, around six to eight sessions for IBS is usually enough. At this time the client is expected to have understood the treatment techniques well enough to continue treatment themselves if necessary. This is very short-term when compared to traditional psychoanalytical treatment that consists of two to three treatment sessions every week for four to five years. For CBT to work, the person must understand the principles behind the therapy. The therapy is unlikely to be successful otherwise.

Box 13. **An example of the basis of CBT treatment as explained by a therapist.**

After taking a detailed history of the problem the therapist explained:

Pain or discomfort in our abdomen, diarrhoea, flatulence and constipation in any combination occurs to most of us in our lifetimes.

- If we experience a particularly nasty bout of symptoms this can make us vulnerable to experiencing these symptoms more and more.
- IBS is not a physical disease,
- It is a problem of how your digestive system functions.
- It cannot kill you and is unlikely to get much worse.
- It normally comes and goes.
- For some people it will go away completely and for others it will never totally get better.

Once we can accept this we can learn to control it. This will make it much easier to live with and may even stop it for good.

It has been demonstrated that IBS is aggravated by stress.

This does not mean that IBS is all in the mind – far from it – IBS may have physical causes, but what we do, think and feel aggravates and maintains many of these physical causes.

IBS is likely to be connected to our lifestyle, our level of anxiety and the way we view the world and the symptoms.

Looking at and modifying what we feel, think and do, will reduce the effects of IBS on us and allow us to lead a less restricted life.

It is OK to have IBS. It is nothing to be ashamed of or apologetic about. However, there are lots of things you can do to reduce the effect it has on you.

There are many different strategies and techniques that may be used in CBT. I have included a manual for CBT of IBS at the end of this chapter (see Box 14) which both therapists and people considering undergoing CBT should find clearly outlines many of them.

CASE STUDY CASE STUDY CASE STUDY CASE STUDY

Undergoing CBT for IBS.

Bunty and her therapist identified the following possible maintaining behaviour: Bunty avoided walking with her boyfriend for fear of being caught short without a public toilet and being incontinent. She had never been incontinent in the past. This restricted her life and affected the relationship with her boyfriend. She agreed to test out her fear and risk walking with her boyfriend without knowing where the toilet was. She subsequently found that, even though she did have some urge to go to the toilet, she was able to control this until reaching a convenient place. By the end of treatment she was able to go into any situation without knowledge of where toilets were located and no longer avoided walking with her boyfriend.

Does it work?

CBT has already been found to be a safe and effective treatment for many disorders such as anxiety and depression and in the last few years there have been an increasing number of studies showing that CBT can be effective for IBS. The *Journal of Consulting Clinical Psychology* published a research study by Greene and Blanchard in 1994 describing the effectiveness of individual cognitive therapy in the treatment of IBS.

Twenty patients with IBS were randomly divided into two groups. One group received 10 individual sessions of psychotherapy over an 8-week period. The second group was instructed to monitor their digestive symptoms. The results showed that, in comparing the symptom picture prior to psychotherapy to that after receiving treatment, the CBT group showed significant reductions in digestive symptoms as compared to the second group. These beneficial results of CBT in IBS were still there when patients were re-evaluated three months later.

A study by one of the present authors and his colleagues (Chalder *et al.*, in press) examined the addition of CBT to standard medical treatment of drug therapy. Specially trained nurses in the patients' GP surgeries provided the CBT. We found that CBT was very effective in reducing symptoms and improving quality of life after treatment and at 6-month follow-up.

The above study used specially trained nurses to deliver the CBT. One of the problems in trying to get CBT for IBS is that therapists are usually in great demand and tend to concentrate on many other disorders than IBS. This can make CBT for IBS difficult to obtain. CBT may not be suitable for IBS if there is associated severe mental illness or drug- or alcohol-dependence.

Scientific research	13
Availability	5
Cost	7 (cost varies but available on the NHS)
Attractiveness	8
Total score	*33*

Box 14. **Therapist guidelines of cognitive behavioural therapy for IBS.**

Clarifying the diagnosis prior to starting CBT

For cognitive behavioural therapy a diagnosis of IBS is not strictly necessary. Rather it is important to have an understanding of the thoughts, feelings and behaviours that occur around the symptoms experienced by the patient. Whether or not the patient has IBS is not the main issue in treatment. The main issue is how the person perceives and copes with the ongoing symptoms such as diarrhoea, bloating and abdominal pain. The ideal situation prior to starting CBT would be one where the patient and GP reach a stage where they have agreed that:

'At our current understanding of these problems, the patient's symptoms have no known cause/pathology at this time',
    and
'the symptoms fluctuate according to what else is happening in the patient's life'.

We would expect patients to experience symptoms associated with IBS after the treatment has been completed. The focus of CBT is the behaviours, thoughts and feelings surrounding the IBS with the aim of improving the way people cope with day-to-day life. Improving these aspects of life we believe will, in turn, reduce the physical symptoms of IBS.

The way a patient thinks, acts and feels can intensify and maintain the symptoms.

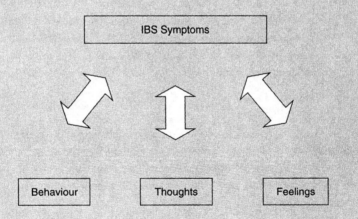

This in turn will affect many aspects of their daily life.

If patients experience a particularly nasty bout of symptoms, this can cause them to focus on the symptoms much more (becoming hypersensitive to them), which then increases the impact and frequency of the IBS symptoms. This is referred to as 'symptoms focusing'. The patient should understand that this does not mean that IBS is all in the mind but rather that, even though IBS may have physical causes that we have yet to discover, what a person does, thinks and feels will aggravate and maintain many of the IBS symptoms.

IBS is likely to be connected to our lifestyle, our level of anxiety and the way we view the world.

During the assessment a therapist should ascertain which thoughts and behaviours are aggravating or maintaining IBS symptoms. Once the patient can understand the CBT model and how it fits with their own experience of IBS, then the therapist should explain how further sessions will aim to lessen the impact of IBS and, in turn, reduce the symptoms.

The therapist should explain to the patient that treatment is collaborative, i.e. the therapist and patient work together to identify possible maintaining factors and test out ways of improving the way they are coping with IBS. The style of therapy is often referred to as 'collaborative empiricism'. Thoughts and behaviours that may be maintaining aspects of the IBS are identified and then alternative behaviours which might be more appropriate are suggested and tested.

The therapist should demonstrate a positive regard for the patient and their problems. The therapist should try and avoid using medical jargon and, where possible, use the patient's language. The therapist will have a good working knowledge of IBS and problems associated with it.

Treatment does not focus on cause and onset. The patient is likely to still have IBS at the end of treatment and they will still have bouts of symptoms. The aim of treatment is to help the patient manage these symptoms in a way that will have minimal effect on their individual lifestyle.

Treatment outline

Between 6 and 9 sessions is usually enough for treatment. Sessions should average 50 minutes and be no longer than 90 minutes. This maximum time encourages therapists to tailor their interventions with the individual patient.
Each session should contain the following components:

- Feedback from previous session.
- Collaborative agenda setting.
- Homework review.
- Homework discussion.
- Goal-setting.
- Recap of key issues.

The treatment sessions should also include the following components, as necessary:

(1) Information-giving about the problems associated with IBS.

(2) Continuing to identify the maintaining factors of IBS.

(3) Introducing IBS-specific behavioural and cognitive strategies.

(4) Checking understanding and acceptance of the treatment rationale.

(5) Using questionnaires as a therapeutic tool to monitor progress.

(6) Encouraging the use of diaries.

First week's goals

Agreeing on the first week's goals is important to the success of treatment. The goals should focus on a small specific behaviour that the person can identify as being a positive step in improving behaviour associated with the IBS, often reinforcing the CBT treatment rationale. For example:

- To spend a maximum of 15 minutes on the toilet each time I go this week.

This goal should have, approximately, an 85 per cent chance of being successfully achieved within the next week. Therapist and patient will check for any possible problems or obstacles that may arise in the completion of this goal and, deal with these or adjust the goal accordingly.

Sometimes it is difficult to agree on long-term problems and targets in the first session. The therapist may suggest that the patient make a list of the goals of therapy before the next session.

Monitoring symptoms and behaviour

For the first week only all patients should be asked to use a diary to monitor their symptom severity, the situations they arise in, and their thoughts and behaviours associated with these symptoms.

The aim of this diary is to gather further information about the day-to-day effects of symptoms and behaviour. This diary will then be used to help construct targets in future sessions.

Therapists should warn patients that focusing on symptoms for the first week may actually cause the symptoms to get worse. This may be used as an example of how focusing causes symptoms to increase. The symptom monitoring will only happen for one week. At the next session the symptom monitoring sheet is reviewed and therapist and patient will then identify and prioritise triggers and agree upon targets for the next week. If possible these should be behavioural targets, either facing previously avoided behaviour or reducing excess precautions or safety behaviour.

Example targets:

(1) Not to read every time I use the toilet.

(2) To use the toilet only when I have a definite urge to pass a stool.

(3) To visit the cinema once a week (or another activity) without using the toilet for 1 hour before.

(4) To eat two slices of toast for breakfast every weekday.

(5) Not to check my stool for abnormalities this week.

(6) Not to carry my IBS medication when going outside this week.

The specific weekly targets chosen will vary according to each individual's needs and circumstances.

The patient is encouraged to take a lead in choosing target behaviours, if possible from the initial diaries. His or her commitment is sought to undertake these targets even when symptomatic, and not to abandon it when symptoms develop, but to continue to practise according to an agreed, pre-set timetable.

Patients may be encouraged to telephone their therapist if they have any difficulties in between sessions. Further sessions will be conducted in a similar manner, making the link between thoughts, feelings and behaviour, with specific strategies for specific symptoms.

The kitbag approach

As specific issues arise, the therapist will identify the specific technique that may be appropriate from a 'therapeutic kitbag'. This is a collection of techniques that have been derived from the cognitive behavioural model but address specific issues that often arise with patients with IBS. The identification of these issues will rely on good communication between patient and therapist as well as on regular clinical supervision.

The kitbag can be divided into five sections:

Section one: Educational advice

Education and advice may be given to change any misconceptions concerning bowel function.

1. Frequency and consistency of stool motion

Examples of misconceptions:

'I should pass a stool every day.'

'Stools must be a certain shape and form.'

The hunt for the perfect stool: some patients will examine each stool that they pass, wanting to achieve a perfect stool that has never been achieved.

Therapists may discuss what affects the frequency and consistency of stools, the role of mood, changing diet, stress, anxiety and worry or change of environment

2. The nature of the digestive system

Examples of misconceptions:

'If I am unable to get rid of all my stool it is dirty/dangerous.'

Therapists should have a working knowledge of the digestive system and how food passes through the body.

3. The role of diet

Examples of misconceptions:

'By avoiding certain food I will avoid/control my symptoms.'

'By avoiding eating at certain times I will avoid/control certain symptoms.'

Some misconceptions will also contain statements that need a more cognitive intervention, e.g. 'should' statements. This approach is outlined below.

4. Misinterpretation of IBS symptoms

Some of the symptoms of IBS are often misinterpreted. An example of symptom misinterpretation is as follows:

Tricia often experiences the feeling of incomplete evacuation (a very common symptom in IBS). When experiencing this symptom she believes she must pass a stool and if she doesn't this will cause her harm or damage. This leads to excessive straining or even occasional manual evacuation in the attempt to reduce this feeling.

During the session it was explained that the feeling of incomplete evacuation is a symptom of IBS and does not mean that the Tricia must pass a stool. Once Tricia understood this, she was advised just to experience the symptom and not react in her previous manner.

She was able to learn to distinguish between this feeling of incomplete evacuation and the actual feeling that she needed to pass a stool.

Section two: Behavioural techniques

Reintroducing avoided foods

Rationale: Often people with IBS may link specific foods and drinks to their symptoms. These are often very idiosyncratic and associations are frequently made after only one bad association, e.g. 'I got the runs after drinking Ribena, and so avoid it totally now'. This can cause moderate to severe limitations on a person's life. Being in treatment is an ideal opportunity to re-test these associations in a systematic way. After re-testing these foods it will be more possible to make a decision about their exclusion from your diet.

Technique: Make a list of avoided foods. Decide which food would be a good starting point, e.g. foods that I would like/should be able/are good for me to eat, foods that I avoid that are inconvenient to the way I would like to live my life. Agree, and set targets for, foods to try during the following two weeks, specifying frequency and amount of food to be eaten. Predict and problem-solve possible problems that may occur.

Reducing toilet behaviour

Rationale: The act of going to the toilet often involves many micro-behaviours that may help maintain IBS symptoms. As with food avoidance, these behaviours need to be assessed and reduced.

Examples of toilet micro-behaviour:

Excessive wiping, checking, or time spent on toilet.

Manual evacuation.

Straining: This is probably the most important of behaviours to assess and reduce. People often strain because they feel they will be unable to pass a stool without it. Often people can strain for long periods of time and still only manage to pass small stools if any at all. Assess the length of time spent straining and severity of the 'push' and agree on how they will reduce this. The aim should be to reduce straining completely by the end of treatment.

Section three: Cognitive techniques

The role of our thoughts and the way they relate to physical illness attributes will already have been discussed as part of the treatment rationale. Cognitive techniques may be introduced as particular misconceptions are identified.

The role of thoughts as maintaining factors in IBS is discussed, their relationship to feelings and behaviour is explored, e.g. there may be misconceptions about bowel habit. It is emphasised that these thoughts can initially be hard to identify. It is explained that they may be distortions of ▶

reality that can influence the perception of, response to and maintenance of symptoms, and can lower mood.

Self-monitoring diaries

Self-monitoring diaries for thoughts are introduced, and their use is explained, reinforcing the feeling/thoughts/behaviour link. Persons are asked to record examples of situations in which they experience an unpleasant emotion or mood change, and to write down, as exactly as possible, what is going through their mind at the time.

People should be prepared for the possibility that recording these thoughts may, by heightening awareness, temporarily increase feelings of depression or increase symptom sensitivity. Persons should be advised, if this occurs, to limit time spent focusing on distressing thoughts.

Once these diaries have been completed, then the therapist and person will use them to identify common themes and thinking errors and then discuss suitable alternatives that may be used instead. This may be done by testing out people's predictions.

Testing out predictions

Examples of predictions persons make:

'Others will notice the smell.'

'I will have an accident if I wait more than one minute.'

'My doctor has missed something that will cause me irrevocable harm.'

'I have a serious illness like bowel cancer.'

The 'for and against' technique

Once the belief is identified, people are asked to list statements that support the belief. They are then asked to rate their strength of belief for each statement. They are then asked to list statements that are against the belief, as well as rating the strength of beliefs for each. They are then asked to reassess their original statements.

Section four: Symptom management techniques

Reducing symptom focusing

Rationale: Bloating and abdominal pain are common symptoms of IBS. By attending to the abdominal areas, people are more likely to have an increased sensitivity to any abdominal change. Once you focus on the symptoms, then you are likely to experience more pain and bloating more and more frequently. By using a range of techniques we can reduce this focusing and thus reduce pain and bloating.

1. Watch out for when you make predictions about the onset of bloating and pain.

Example of symptom focusing:

'I have just eaten a cheese roll, that's going to give me hell!'

Once we have these types of thoughts we are more likely to focus on the abdominal area. This will make us more sensitive to any changes that may have occurred anyway. Once we have felt a change we are more likely to have think, 'Oh no, I can feel it starting, its getting worse, I can't control this'. This increases our focusing on the area and is more likely to increase the symptoms.

2. Be aware when you are focusing, do not ignore the pain, but carry on with it.

3. Be aware of your thoughts when you first become aware of the symptoms.

The 'getting a second head' technique

Rationale: We have found that this is something that people often find helpful when the symptoms get on top of them. Recognise when you need to do this. Try and step out of your head and look at your symptoms from another perspective.

It is the difference between 'I am not coping with it all' to 'I am having thoughts about not coping with my IBS'.

The first, 'I am not coping with it all', will naturally make us feel worse: it does not allow us to do anything about it; it's a dead-end statement.

See your thoughts, don't **be** your thoughts.

Accepting the IBS

Rationale: This sounds easy to say but it is very important in the reduction of symptoms. What do you say to yourself when you get symptoms of IBS? If you think, 'Oh my God, I've started to feel bloated, it's bound to get worse and then ruin my night out', this is more likely to lead to increased worry, stress and focusing on the bloating. The way we think about our IBS will affect our symptoms. Recognise when this is happening and challenge those ▶

thoughts, e.g. 'OK, I have bloating, but I have had it this bad before, I will still go out and make the most of my night out. I will not let the IBS rule me. By still going out I will be in control.'

Section five: Mixed techniques

Special diets and food intake

Special diets have been shown to be of little benefit. It was thought, for example, that a high-fibre diet was beneficial, but recent studies have shown that this is not necessary. It is important, however, that the person does not become too obsessed with diet, otherwise their eating habits may be governed by fear that the discomfort or pain may return.

Constantly fluctuating diet will lead to fluctuating pain and discomfort.

It is important to stabilise the person's diet during treatment. This will allow you and the person to evaluate any changes made as a result of the therapy and not anything else. A constant regular diet may also help reduce some of the IBS symptoms.

Healthy bowel routine

The following is a list of basic guidelines to facilitate a healthy bowel routine:

(1) Eat at regular hours; chew food slowly and thoroughly.

(2) Drink two litres of liquid daily, including fruit and vegetable juices and water.

(3) Maintain a regular programme of physical exercise and activity. We suggest walking three times a week for a minimum of 30 minutes.

(4) Always act on the urge to have a bowel movement.

(5) Avoid straining.

The use of a key card

The idea that symptoms will continue to arise from time to time should be reinforced, and it should be stressed that the person can deal with them effectively. People are encouraged to write a list of what they have learned/found most useful in treatment and to plan mini-programmes to deal with potential setbacks. This 'key card' can be used as a reminder and prompt when problems arise in the future.

We would like to acknowledge the contribution of Trudie Chalder and Tom Kennedy to the preparation of this manual.

Summary

- Psychological treatments can help people with severe chronic IBS. People with mild IBS do not need psychological treatment.

- It does not mean that IBS is all in the mind. It is not!

- Psychological treatments are unlikely to remove IBS totally but can improve many of the symptoms and make life a lot more bearable.

- Gut-directed hypnotherapy is very effective; but beware of other forms of hypnotherapy.

- Dynamic psychotherapy may be of some help, but can be costly and time-consuming.

- Cognitive behavioural therapy can also be useful, but can be difficult to access.

- Always check the qualifications and experience of the therapist.

Other alternative treatments

6

The aim of this chapter is to review the range of complementary therapies that people with IBS may have recourse to.

Bookshop and library shelves groan and buckle as they struggle to support the ever-increasing wealth of literature available on the burgeoning number of complementary (also known as alternative) therapies now practised in the UK.

Whatever you may wish to discover – from how the healing power of rose quartz, amethyst or other semi-precious stones can be harnessed through gem therapy, to how Kirlian photography records a person's electromagnetic 'aura' to determine potential health hazards – there will be a book, or three, about it.

Trying to find out what complementary therapies *may* work for IBS, however, can prove to be a bit of a minefield. The fluctuating nature of the condition means that almost every form of therapy known has, at some point, claimed success in treating IBS.

The complementary therapies described below have each been given scores out of 50 for scientific research, availability, cost and attractiveness (see Chapter 5, p. 61, for the explanation of the scoring).

Acupuncture

Acupuncture is an ancient Chinese medical procedure involving insertion and manipulation of needles at more than 360 points – known as acupoints – in the body. The treatment has been said to relieve symptoms of some physical and psychological conditions and may encourage the body to heal and repair itself.

In Traditional Chinese Medicine, it is believed an energy called 'chi' flows along invisible energy channels called 'meridians', which are believed to be linked to internal organs. Sticking needles at particular points along these meridians is believed to increase or decrease the flow of energy. Fine needles are inserted through the skin and left in position briefly, sometimes with manual or electrical stimulation. The number of needles varies, but it may be only two or three. Acupuncture stimulates the nerves in skin and muscle, which is claimed to increase the body's release of natural painkillers – endorphin and serotonin – and to modify the way pain signals are received.

A small cone of powdered 'moxa', a drug derived from the dried herb lugwort, may also be applied to an acupoint. This is then ignited, which is designed to warm and stimulate the chi. This is known as moxibustion.

Acupuncturists claim that patients often notice an improved sense of well-being after treatment, as well as a reduction in pain. Each patient's case will be assessed by the practitioner and treatment tailored to the individual. Treatment might be once a week to begin with, then at longer intervals as the condition responds.

Acupuncture has been used for digestive problems such as IBS. It is also claimed to help with stopping smoking. Acupuncture-like techniques have been used for over 5000 years, initially developed in the Far East and then introduced into Europe in the seventeenth century. However, widespread interest in the technique did not develop until the 1970s, when travel restrictions between the East and the West were eased.

In the past 30 years some scientific research has been carried out on acupuncture, although there is still much more to be done. It is now, however, accepted by many in the orthodox medical establishment. The technique is now used alongside conventional medicine, in a number of hospital pain clinics and by an increasing number of GPs, hospital doctors and physiotherapists. However, most practice a 'Westernised' form of acupuncture, which does not use the traditional Chinese medicine philosophy.

Scientific research	8
Availability	5
Cost	4
Attractiveness	7
Total score	*24*

Acupressure

Acupressure is a variant of acupuncture in which the practitioner uses manipulation, rather than penetration, to alleviate pain or other symptoms. It is in widespread use in Japan and popular also in the United States and elsewhere. Also known as 'shiatsu', acupressure is administered by pressing with the fingertips – and sometimes the elbows and knees – along a complex network of trigger points in the patient's body. There have been no studies to determine the success of this treatment for IBS.

Scientific research	6
Availability	3
Cost	4
Attractiveness	7
Total score	*20*

Alexander technique

The Alexander technique is a method of bringing the way we move under conscious control and avoiding build-up of muscular tension. By learning to stand correctly it is claimed that stresses on the body are eased and complaints that are exacerbated by poor posture are alleviated. Alexander technique teachers help to adjust the client's posture and, by means of verbal instruction and postural guidance, teach people how to become more aware of their posture, balance and movement in everyday life. The technique is based on the principle that the mind and body are inextricably linked and that, by influencing one, it is possible to have a profound effect on the other.

The lessons usually last for 30–45 minutes on a one-to-one basis, the teacher using their hands to correct any muscular imbalances, encouraging the body to a better alignment. Alexander technique teachers say that this process of re-educating the body by learning how to stand and move correctly leads to health benefits as, often, poor spinal posture will cause other symptoms. Breathing problems can be improved and stress-related symptoms reduced, they say. The technique was developed at the turn of the twentieth century by an Australian actor, Frederick Mathias Alexander, who claimed to have restored his own health and then taught others to do the same.

Scientific research	4
Availability	3
Cost	4/5
Attractiveness	7
Total score	*19*

Applied kinesiology

Applied kinesiology uses muscle testing, which is claimed to detect imbalances in body systems and sensitivities to food and toxic substances in the environment.

It is a system of diagnosis used by some chiropractors, homeopaths, naturopaths and nutrition therapists. The method works on the theory that foods or chemicals to which an individual is sensitive cause muscle weakening as a result of their changing the body's electrical field. Practitioners place suspect substances in the patient's hand or under their tongue and check for muscle weakening by pressing against it while the patient holds steady. If the limb sags or feels 'spongy' they say this indicates an imbalance. Further tests are carried out to find out why and the patient is treated accordingly. There is absolutely no specific research on the applicability of kinesiology for IBS.

Scientific research	2
Availability	2
Cost	5
Attractiveness	7
Total score	*16*

Aromatherapy

Aromatherapy, the practice of using pure essential oils, derived from plants, either in combination or on their own, to treat ailments has its roots back in ancient Egypt. In 1937 the term 'aromatherapy' was used by a French chemist in a book which described the healing powers of essential oils. The practice was also used on wounded soldiers by a French surgeon in World War II. Robert Tisserand brought aromatherapy to Britain in the late 1960s and opened the first training institute in the UK.

Aromatherapy – the fastest-growing of all complementary therapies – works on the principle that certain aromas, or smells, can have a positive influence on health, with specific aromas being most effective against specific conditions. Aromatherapy is claimed to stimulate the brain, releasing neurotransmitters, which have a far-reaching effect on all levels of function. It is often used in the NHS and in private hospitals and hospices.

The aromatherapist attempts, through questioning, to understand what is 'wrong' with a patient and then identifies the blend of essential oils required to alleviate that problem. Essential oils are blended with a carrier oil, such as almond oil, for the purposes of massage. Pure essential oils are never put directly onto the skin. While it takes a lengthy training period to become a qualified aromatherapist, oils can be purchased for some simpler, self-care applications or to improve general well-being. People often say that aromatherapy is great but that it has not necessarily improved their IBS. Aromatherapists, however, believe that essential oils have a deeper medicinal value, maintaining that some oils have anti-inflammatory properties, others are good for the intestines and yet others will help to reduce mucus.

Scientific research	4
Availability	8
Cost	4
Attractiveness	8
Total score	*24*

Ayurveda

Ayurveda claims to be probably the most ancient of all medical systems. Historical records have revealed that Ayurvedic hospitals were being built by ancient Sri Lankan kings as far back as 437 BC. It is said that one king even constructed 18 state-funded Ayurvedic hospitals, starting from 161 BC, and it is still the most important form of medicine in the Indian subcontinent. Training takes a very long time and the philosophy of the system is extremely complex. Classical Ayurvedic training is conducted in Sanskrit. Most Ayurvedic practitioners tend to be orthodox doctors as well.

The word 'Ayurveda' comes from Sanskrit and means 'the science of life'. Central to the concept of Ayurveda is the concept of 'psycho-biological individuality' – the notion that every person is a unique individual, not just in terms of personality but also their specific type of bodily constitution, known as the 'prakriti'. The whole aim of Ayurveda is prevention. The Ayurvedic practitioner aims to balance the body and mind, find health problems before they occur or arrest them before they do any real harm. It is a complete philosophical and spiritual system. Ayurvedic philosophy believes that emotional repression can lead to illnesses such as IBS, through the production and build-up of toxins in the body. Ayurvedic medicine is offered as a treatment for IBS.

The five elements – ether, air, fire, water and earth – are the foundations on which the Ayurvedic interpretation of all matter and life is based. Each represents qualities and different types of force and energy, as well as some form of physical manifestation. It is believed that these elements do not act in isolation – three different combinations of the elements, called 'doshas', form the basis for diagnosis, treatment, cure and health maintenance by Ayurvedic practitioners. Each individual's body type is determined at birth when each person has the levels of the three doshas that is right for them. Life and all its forces can cause the doshas to become unbalanced and that can lead to ill-health.

Each of the three doshas has a role to play in the body:

- *Vatha* relates to movement, including respiration, circulation and the nervous system. Vatha imbalances are associated with diseases of the nervous system, chronic pain, rheumatic problems, constipation, anxiety and insomnia.
- *Pitta* affects metabolic activity, especially the digestive system. Problems associated with pitta imbalances include peptic ulcers, dermatitis and other skin allergies, hypertension and bowel diseases.
- *Kapha* governs the structure and fluid balance of the body. Diabetes, asthma, hayfever and depression can result from kapha imbalances.

There is no typical Ayurvedic session – even the methods of diagnosis may differ from practitioner to practitioner. After diagnosis comes treatment and the range of treatments is vast, including guidelines for healthy living and diet instructions. Other healing techniques including massage, exercise and breathing, and meditation may also be offered.

Scientific research	0
Availability	3
Cost	5
Attractiveness	6
Total score	*14*

Biofeedback

Biofeedback is described as a relaxation technique for learning to control a bodily function that is not normally under conscious control, such as skin temperature, blood pressure or muscle tension. It is claimed that biofeedback techniques can be used to manage IBS. Biofeedback training may help to relieve pain from intestinal spasms and also may help to improve bowel movement control in people who have severe diarrhoea.

It is a painless process that uses a computer and a video monitor to display bodily functions that we are usually not aware of. Special sensors measure these functions, which are displayed as sounds or as line graphs on the computer. A therapist helps clients to use this information to modify or change abnormal responses to more normal patterns.

Biofeedback practitioners claims that bowel control is a bodily function that can be shaped by the technology by allowing clients to retrain 'defective processes' and to restore more normal functions.

Scientific research   6

Availability   3

Cost   2

Attractiveness   5

Total score   16

Breathing and relaxation

Proper breathing and the ability to relax have been described as essential aspects of dealing with stress. The importance of relaxation and proper breathing is recognised by many complementary health practitioners and their practice has been the core, for hundreds of years, of many Eastern philosophies and is now practised more and more in the West. Breathing exercises and relaxation techniques, such as 'progressive muscular relaxation', works by initiating the 'relaxation response', a physiological mechanism which counteracts the effects of stress and puts mind and body into a profound state of relaxation. This has been promoted as a good way of coping with IBS. Conventional medicine is increasingly valuing the health benefits of breathing and relaxation techniques and they are often taught in hospitals and health centres. The teaching can take place in groups or on an individual basis.

T'ai chi

T'ai chi, is often described as martial arts without the violence. It is an ancient system of oriental medicine which combines a gentle martial art with meditation and a series of exercises said to enhance the health of the body and mind. It is also practised as a form of relaxation. It incorporates other Chinese therapies, including acupuncture and herbal medicine, and is claimed to be a powerful way to combat stress and ease stress-related disorders such as IBS.

Scientific research   6

Availability   9

Cost   1–7 (varies)

Attractiveness   7

Total score   29

Relaxation is so common – yet it has never fully proved itself as an effective treatment for IBS, although many people say they find it useful and many really like the effects in the short-term.

❝I did find it relaxing – it made me fall asleep.❞

❝My doctor gave me one of those relaxation tapes ... it was good ... but the problem was I never got round to using it often ... I can't seem to find the time.❞

Although relaxation tapes are undoubtedly good for some people, many have found it difficult deliberately to try to relax.

❝I concentrated so hard on trying to relax that it just made me more tense.❞

❝As the time drew near to do my relaxation, I began to worry ... while doing it I was worried that I might not be doing it right.❞

Have a look at your daily life and what it is that you find relaxing – perhaps it is keeping up to date with the daily newspaper or becoming engrossed in a good novel, wallowing in a long, hot soak in the bath, pottering round the garden, catching up with an old friend on the telephone, indulging in a hobby or simply blobbing out on the sofa in front of a trashy TV programme. Our lives are so busy we often find it difficult to do these things as often as we should. The key is to make time for them – at least one hour a day should be spent on an utterly relaxing activity.

Colonic irrigation

Colonic irrigation is also known as 'colonic hydrotherapy' or 'colon therapy' and was reputedly used in ancient Egypt, China and India. However, the method common in the West today has its origins in nineteenth-century European spas and involves washing out the large intestine, a sort of 'internal bath'. Some IBS sufferers are known to use the practice, although it has not been the subject of any specific trials for IBS so far.

A treatment will begin with a detailed case study, and an explanation of the procedure. The client is then asked to remove all clothing and wear a gown provided by the therapist. The client then lies down on a treatment table and warm, purified water is introduced into the colon via the rectum. The therapist will use massage techniques during the procedure to stimulate the release of stored faecal matter. The treatment will take between 30 and 45 minutes. Herbal and probiotic implants may be used and advice given on dietary changes to enhance the treatment. A colon-cleansing programme may be recommended to support the treatment.

Scientific research	0
Availability	7
Cost	6
Attractiveness	3
Total score	*16*

Herbal medicine

Herbal medicine is one of the oldest therapies of all. Early records show that the Egyptians used herbal medicine as far back as the sixteenth century BC. The Greek 'father of medicine', Hippocrates, also had a significant impact on the burgeoning use of herbs, practising a system of holistic medicine focusing on the person, rather than on the disease. Herbalism is still the most widely practised form of medicine in the world today, with over 80 per cent of the planet's population relying on herbs for health.

Many of the pharmaceutical drugs used today are derived from herbs, for instance *acetylsalicylic acid*, or *aspirin*, originally derived from willow-tree bark, and the heart drug *digitalis* which comes from foxgloves. However, these drugs are based on what are considered to be the plant's 'active' ingredients – that is, certain chemicals that have been isolated from the original plant – whereas herbalism utilises the whole plant or, at the very least, the seed, root or flower.

Herbalists believe that the body has its own ability to heal itself. Herbs can help support this system, enabling balance to be restored to the body. Herbs are administered in many ways and are used both internally and topically. Some herbs, such as mint, ginger, chamomile, fennel, dandelion, peppermint and aloe vera have been used to in an attempt to alleviate some of the symptoms of IBS. Meadowsweet, marshmallow root, bayberry, slippery elm and comfrey may all be used to reduce irritability in the wall of the intestine. Linseed may be prescribed for constipation and liquorice is another powerful anti-inflammatory which also has laxative qualities. Herbalists use it in very small doses.

A recent, high-quality, randomised trial of Chinese herbal medicine has provided good evidence for its effectiveness in treating IBS (Bensoussan *et al.*, 1998). The trial, probably the first to have adhered both to the principles of Chinese herbal medicine and to accepted principles of methodological rigour, gave a group of people with IBS either a placebo or standard or individualised Chinese herbal medicine. The triallists went to a great deal of trouble to ensure the high standard of the study. They ensured that the herbal medicines used both for standard treatment and for individualised treatment came from a common Chinese herbal pharmacopoeia. They ensured that the placebo was similar in taste and appearance to the Chinese herbal medicine. They used a standard diagnosis for IBS and standard scales for IBS symptoms and severity. Finally, patient and gastroenterologist scored independently.

Patients were randomised and then saw their herbal practitioner at two-week intervals for two occasions and then monthly for a further two occasions, with continuous treatment for 16 weeks in all. At the end of the 16 weeks there was a rating of success (improved, same, worse) by patient and gastroenterologist. At the end of 16 weeks, 29 out of 38 patients judged their IBS to have improved on standard treatment, 18 out of 28 on individualised treatment and 11 out of 33 on placebo. The result was positive – not just positive but with high levels of statistical significance.

Scientific research	14
Availability	5
Cost	2–9 (can vary greatly, shop around)
Attractiveness	6 (the taste can often be disgusting)
Total score	*34*

Homeopathy

Homeopathy is another ancient system of medicine, dating back to the fifth century BC, and resurrected and popularised in the eighteenth century by German physician-chemist Samuel Hahnemann. It is also well known in the UK because of the Royal Family's much-publicised use of it. Homeopathy is a holistic therapy using remedies made from plant, mineral and animal substances in a variety of dilutions to cure a person's illness. It is based on the theory that 'like cures like'. This means that a substance that causes symptoms of illness in a healthy person could be used to treat the same symptoms in someone who is ill.

Substances are diluted many times to make a remedy that is safe to use, but sufficient 'likeness' remains between the remedy and the illness which, say practitioners, will stimulate the body's self-healing abilities, much in the same way as vaccination. Homeopathy treats the whole person and their mental and emotional state, as well as physical symptoms. Homeopathic remedies are prescribed according to each individual's symptom picture, rather than to the illness itself. Thus, different persons suffering the same illness might be given different remedies. There are a number of NHS homeopathic hospitals and a demand for homeopathic remedies is growing.

For IBS sufferers, *ignatia* may be prescribed for spasms of abdominal pain and diarrhoea after emotional upsets. For those who suffer from pain which is relieved by passing wind and whose stools are bulky and may contain mucus, *graphites* may be offered. A person who suffers from sudden, cramp-like pains which are made worse by eating and drinking may respond to *colocynthis*.

Scientific research	2
Availability	9
Cost	6 (varies)
Attractiveness	8
Total score	*25*

Manual lymphatic drainage

Manual lymphatic drainage is a gentle, rhythmic massage that is said to stimulate the lymphatic vessels leading to the re-absorption and removal of excess metabolic waste, debris and toxins from the body tissues. Lymph moves water, protein, white blood cells and electrolytes around the body, beneath the skin. The greater the flow of lymph, it is said, the healthier the body will be. Practitioners say that manual lymphatic drainage can help move the excess fluid from the tissues and the accompanying relief of fluid congestion promotes healing, strengthens the immune system and can reduce pain. It also claims to be extremely relaxing and rejuvenating and to have been successfully used to treat IBS.

Scientific research	0
Availability	2
Cost	7
Attractiveness	8
Total score	*17*

Metabolic typing

Metabolic typing is, in short, 'customised nutrition', based on the idea that there is no universal healthy diet to suit everyone. Anyone can use metabolic typing to find out exactly which foods are good for their health and those that are not. It is a way of evaluating the interrelationship of the body's three main systems for the creation and maintenance of energy – the autonomic nervous system, the oxidative system and the endocrine system. Practitioners say that no adverse condition can exist without a metabolic imbalance in one or more of these systems. They add that these metabolic imbalances are very common and most people who are chronically unwell have at least one of them. When a person is 'balanced' metabolically, it is claimed that many disease symptoms subside because the body uses nutrients optimally.

Scientific research   2

Availability   4

Cost   3–8 (varies)

Attractiveness   6 (sometimes difficult to follow regime)

Total score   *20*

Naturopathy

Naturopathy or 'naturopathic medicine' is not a technique but a system of natural healthcare that believes the body has the knowledge to heal itself. Naturopaths see illness as evidence that a body is not in harmony and perfect balance with the environment. The treatment they provide addresses the underlying causes of illness, primarily unfavourable lifestyle habits. Naturopaths claim to facilitate the process of the body healing itself with the aid of natural, non-toxic therapies. The term 'naturopath' was coined by a German homeopath, John H. Scheel, to denote health promotion and the treatment of the whole person with natural means. A naturopath will often view themselves as a teacher, whose job is to educate and support the client.

Diet is probably the most important aspect in naturopathy and is designed to strengthen the body or free it from toxins or allergens. Most naturopathic diets focus on wholefoods and vegetarian organic foods, eaten in their raw state. Patients may be advised to go on a complete or partial fast for up to seven days at a time.

The treatment can also include: physiotherapy, therapeutic exercise, reflexology, acupuncture, hydrotherapies, biofeedback, meditation, nutrition, herbal remedies, homeopathic remedies. Naturopathy can be used to treat a wide variety of illnesses and complaints and IBS sufferers may benefit. However, treatment is often dictated by the patient's willingness to change or participate.

Scientific research   4

Availability   4

Cost   4–9 (varies)

Attractiveness   6

Total score   *19*

Polarity therapy

Polarity therapy, developed by Dr Randolph Stone in the late nineteenth century, is a blend of Western therapies, traditional Chinese medicine and Ayurveda. Well-being is said to be the result of the unobstructed flow of the 'life force' around the body. This life force corresponds to 'chi' or 'Qi' in traditional Chinese medicine and 'Prana' in Ayurveda. This life force or energy is thought to move in currents around the body between positive and negative poles. Practitioners aim to rebalance or restore the energy flow by means of bodywork, nutritional advice, gentle stretching exercises – polarity yoga – and counselling.

Scientific research	0
Availability	4
Cost	3–8
Attractiveness	3
Total score	*15*

Probiotics

Probiotics are micro-organisms that help maintain the natural balance of organisms (microflora) in the intestines. The normal human digestive tract contains about 400 types of normal bacteria which reduce the growth of harmful bacteria and promote a healthy digestive system. The largest group of probiotic bacteria in the intestine is lactic acid bacteria of which *Lactobacillus acidophilus*, found in yoghurt, is the best-known. Yeast is also a probiotic substance.

Beneficial bacteria often are used to replace normal bacteria that are lost after a person takes antibiotics to treat an infection. Antibiotics kill susceptible bacteria along with the bacteria that cause illness. This can lead to the development of other infections, such as candida and urinary tract infections, and symptoms such as diarrhoea from intestinal illnesses. Taking probiotic substances (in capsule, powder or liquid form) may help to replace the lost beneficial bacteria. Probiotics might improve constipation or diarrhoea caused by IBS but more studies are needed to confirm or deny these benefits.

Scientific research	0
Availability	3
Cost	4–6
Attractiveness	5
Total score	*14*

Reflexology

Reflexology is claimed to be much more than just a foot massage. It is a complementary therapy, practitioners say, that works on the feet to enable the body to heal itself. It is said to be able to boost energy levels, aid relaxation and stimulate the circulatory system and the body's elimination processes to help with a range of conditions. Reflexology is a treatment which, like acupuncture and acupressure, follows the principle that energy travels through the body along pathways known as meridians or zones, which relate to all the major organs and structures of the body and which are mirrored or 'reflected' on the feet and hands. It was introduced into Britain in the 1960s by Doreen Bayley.

There are ten meridians or zones on the feet and hands (five on each), representing the right and left sides of the body. Within each zone are reflex points along the way. Each zone is associated to a particular organ or structure – liver, heart, bladder, large and small intestine, etc. A reflexologist uses hands only to apply pressure to the feet. Practitioners claim to be able to detect tiny deposits and imbalances in the feet and, by working on these points, reflexologists say they can release blockages and restore the free flow of energy to the whole body.

It has been claimed to be effective at dealing with stress-related conditions such as IBS. However, a study reported in the *British Journal of General Practice*, carried out by Philip Tovey (2002) at the School for Healthcare Studies, Leeds University, investigated the effectiveness of reflexology in treating IBS in four general practices and concluded that there was no evidence, in this particular trial, that reflexology provided any specific benefit for patients with IBS.

Scientific research	0
Availability	6
Cost	4–7 (varies)
Attractiveness	7
Total score	*20*

Thai yoga massage

Thai yoga massage is a mix of both Chinese and Ayurvedic healing systems. The hands, feet and elbows are used to massage energy channels and acupoints along the body, along which prana, the 'life force', is thought to travel, equivalent to the meridians in traditional Chinese medicine. Treatment involves stretching, bending and pulling, intended to restore or improve the flow of prana. In the process a trance-like state is induced which practitioners believe is beneficial for healing.

Scientific research	2
Availability	4
Cost	6–9 (can be expensive)

and meditation in a bid to obtain a harmony of mind, body and spirit. It is not a religion, but a holistic system of therapy that maintains, like Chinese medicine, that illness comes about in the body and mind as a result of imbalances in the 'life force'. The discipline of breathing and concentration during practice is said to bring about a number of benefits which include:

- Increased oxygenation of the blood.
- Muscle toning throughout the body.
- A clearer, more relaxed mind.
- Improved posture.
- Improved circulation of blood and lymph.
- Regulation of bodily functions.

Yoga has been claimed to have a beneficial effect for many sufferers of IBS. There are a variety of yoga styles, which include:

- *Astanga* – a set sequence of postures that will not vary from class to class. The sequences moves through a primary, secondary and advanced series. It is not a beginner's method as some knowledge of postures and their correct form is needed.
- *Bikram* – a form of yoga that teaches 26 postures in a set sequence in a room heated to about 38 degrees Celsius. It is suitable for the beginner or advanced student as the same pattern is always followed. The aim of the class is mostly physical improvement.
- *Hatha* – the basis of most yoga classes. Its aim is to balance people both physically and mentally and to leave you feeling stimulated and relaxed. It is suitable for both beginners and advanced students.
- *Iyengar* – a very thorough form of yoga. The emphasis in class is on correct alignment and the class is suitable for beginners as it helps them to learn each 'asana' or posture.
- *Kundalini* – said to be the most 'spiritual' of the yoga disciplines.
- *Power yoga* – similar to astanga yoga, this form was developed in the United States recently to offer a tough cardio workout. There is no set routine.
- *Sivananda* – this form may use 'mantras' (chanted sounds) and meditation. It is based on 12 basic hatha postures and has a strong emphasis on breathing technique. Much of a class will also be devoted to relaxation.
- *Viniyoga* – a specific one-to-one form of yoga that aims to address individual physical and mental needs.

Attractiveness   6 (can be painful)

Total score   *21*

Traditional Chinese medicine

Traditional Chinese medicine is some 2000 years old. It is based on the principle of internal balance and harmony, 'chi' or 'life force', 'yin' and 'yang' and the five elements. The chi is regulated through meridians or 'energy channels' by the interdependent forces of yin (female) energy and yang (male) energy. It is the job of the practitioner to bring yin and yang back into balance and so regulate the flow of chi through the system, restoring health and harmony.

Chinese herbal medicine

Chinese herbal medicine is a form of traditional Chinese medicine that employs the properties of herbs to prevent and treat physical, mental and emotional ill-health. It may be used alone, or in combination with other therapies. Chinese herbal medicine has been proved to be particularly effective at treating skin disorders, but it is also frequently used for digestive complaints.

Qi Gong

Qi Gong is a component of traditional Chinese medicine and literally means 'energy movement'. Breathing techniques and meditation are used to develop and improve the Qi (chi) or 'life force' around the body. It is believed that these practices help the body and mind to function at optimal levels, increasing vitality and encouraging self-healing.

Scientific research   16

Availability   7

Cost   2–8 (varies)

Attractiveness   5 (again, can taste disgusting)

Total score   *36*

Yoga

Yoga is an ancient Indian system of health developed over 5000 years, using phys-ical postures ('asanas'), breathing exercises ('pranayama'), relaxation techniques

Scientific research	4
Availability	7
Cost	3–7 (varies)
Attractiveness	8
Total score	*26*

Conclusion

Around one-quarter of people in Britain have used sources of healing beyond the realms of recognised conventional treatment at some point in their lives. Over four million visits are now paid, every year, to practitioners of complementary therapies. It clearly has something of offer. But what?

Complementary therapies cover a broad area, embracing Eastern philosophies, manipulative techniques and physical exercises. Some are genuine alternatives to conventional medicine; others remain experimental, even questionable.

Some therapies have been around for thousands of years, others are comparatively new. Some complementary practitioners are highly qualified and highly skilled, some may have been at an evening class or on a weekend course, and some have been known to give themselves imaginary qualifications by using meaningless letters after their name. Some therapies are governed by regulatory bodies, which enforce stringent codes of conduct and provide indemnity should anything go wrong; others are not regulated at all.

Under the rules of science, people who make therapeutic claims for any treatment must conduct suitable studies and report them in detail, to allow evaluation and confirmation by external sources. Conventional medicine does this well. Some complementary therapies, on the other hand, may rely totally on anecdotes and personal testimonies to promote their practices, with no scientific rigour employed whatsoever. And, despite the generally harmless image of complementary therapies, there are risks. Although most problems have been relatively trivial and short-lived, there have been cases of severe injury, infection, allergic reaction and psychological damage as a result of some practices. Any risks, however, can be reduced by ensuring that only a reliable, properly qualified and indemnified practitioner is used – and it is helpful to let GPs know if complementary therapies are being used alongside conventional treatment.

Britain's first-ever Chair in Complementary Medicine has been set up at Exeter University, under the auspices of Professor Edzard Ernst, whose task is to evaluate its scientific validity and safety. Undoubtedly, more and more rigorous studies will be undertaken, ultimately giving the seal of approval to – or rejecting out of hand – the claims made on behalf of the various alternative therapies. Until these studies are carried out, however, complementary therapies perhaps should best be regarded, not as a cure, but as a form of physical, emotional or spiritual support for people who simply wish to feel better.

Summary

- Complementary therapies generally are quite gentle treatments – though this does not apply to them all.

- The patient tends to be in control of the treatment and is able to spend more time with the therapist than would be usual with their doctor.

- The philosophy of complementary therapies is that a person's emotional, physical and spiritual being should remain in balance and harmony at all times.

- Complementary therapists are more likely than orthodox doctors to treat different patients with the same condition differently, the treatment being tailored to individual needs.

- However, many complementary therapies use anecdotal results to suggest the treatment provided is effective. Little scientific research has been done and many of these treatments try to treat the stress associated with IBS, rather than the IBS itself.

- Beware of complementary therapists telling you they can 'cure' your IBS. This has not been demonstrated anywhere, by anybody. Often these treatments are very useful for many people – but they are not a cure.

Jargon busting

Some of the more technical terminology used in discussing IBS is made plain in this chapter, which concludes with a concise summary of the message of this book for IBS sufferers.

Many doctors have been around other doctors too long. As in any profession they will develop their own language or jargon to describe what is happening with their patients. Unfortunately most of us are not doctors (nor would we want to be, given their workload and the increasing state of the NHS). Sometimes, and not deliberately, they forget to translate their jargon back into plain simple English that we all can understand. If a doctor uses a word you do not understand please ask them what they mean. They will not be offended or think you are stupid (unless of course you are a Professor of Medicine, in which case you should know better).

If, however, you are nervous or the jargon was in a written article, then the list below should help decipher what they meant.

Jargon busting list

Anus – the bottom opening of the gut
Abdomen – the area around your tummy and stomach
Abdominal – anything to do with the area around your tummy and stomach
Abdominal distension – where your stomach and tummy actually is sticking out, and you feel full or bloated
Bowel – the bottom part of your guts. It is actually made up of the small and large intestines
Bran – part of cereal grain; it is a great source of fibre
Bulking agent – a treatment given that when swallowed will make your stools bigger, softer and easier to pass; it is often made up of fibre (e.g. Fybogel)
Call to stool – the feeling you have to go for a bowel movement immediately
Colic – spasms in the stomach area causing severe pains
Colectomy – removal of the colon by surgery

Colitis – inflammation of the colon

Colonoscopy – an examination of the colon using a miniature camera or telescope

Constipation – difficulty or straining to pass stools

Crohn's disease – chronic inflammation of part of the alimentary canal of unknown cause

Defecation – the process of passing a stool or motion; going to the toilet

Diarrhoea – passing very loose, watery stools

ENS – (enteric nervous system) a bundle of nerves in the guts that control the intestine functions

Faeces – another word for stools or shit

Familial – something that runs in the family

Flatulence – increased wind or belching

Flatus – wind; farts

Fibre – part of plants that are not digested by the gut

Gastrointestinal – anything around the subject of digestion

Gastroenterologist – a doctor specialising in the area of digestion and bowel disorders

Idiopathic – a condition for which there is no identifiable cause

Intermittent pain – a pain that varies in intensity from time to time

Intestinal transit – the movement of food through the gut

Incontinence – involuntary stool movement (or urine)

Lactose – a type of sugar found in milk

Laxative – a medicine that makes stools softer and easier to pass

Micturition – passing urine

Motility – the time taken for food to pass through your guts, from beginning to end

Mucus – a slimy, jelly-like substance sometimes passed in IBS

Nausea – feeling sick (this does not mean you are always actually sick)

Proctitis – inflammation of the rectum

Rectum – the last bit of the bowel

Refractory – something that does not respond to treatment

Sigmoid – the part of the colon above the rectum

Sigmoidoscopy – a test to look at the sigmoid

Spasm – a rapid contraction of muscles

Syndrome – a set of symptoms

Final words

Irritable bowel syndrome is a pain; it has many difficult and worrying symptoms but, luckily, for most people they will come and go. There are many things still to be discovered about IBS. We do know that some people's bowels are more sensitive than others'. IBS cannot kill you and is unlikely to get much worse. Understanding IBS is the first step to beating it.

We know many things can make IBS worse, for example stress or certain foods, and that drugs and other therapies may help manage the problem. Unfortunately, no one has yet found the cure for IBS. Accepting that you have IBS and coming to terms with it is the second step to beating it.

IBS can, if we let it, affect all areas of our lives. The third step to beating IBS is not to let it stop you from having a good and enjoyable life. Remember, it is OK to have IBS. It is nothing to be ashamed or apologetic about.

Useful addresses

Digestive Disorders Foundation

This is a national charity that is concerned not just with irritable bowel syndrome but the whole range of bowel and digestive problems. They support research at hospitals and universities around the country to improve understanding and develop new treatments.

Digestive Disorders Foundation
PO Box 251
Edgware
Middlesex HA8 6HG

The IBS Network

A UK national charity offering advice, information and support to people with Irritable Bowel Syndrome.

IBS Network
Northern General Hospital
Sheffield
S5 7AU
http://www.ibsnetwork.org.uk
Tel 0114 2611531 Fax 0114 261 0112
e mail penny@ibsnetwork.org.uk
IBS Helpline (calls answered by specialist IBS nurses)
01543 492 192 Monday to Friday 6pm to 8pm
This line is also open on Saturday Morning 10–12 noon

Hypnotherapy

The British Society of Medical and Dental Hypnosis
c/o 42 Links Road
Ashtead
Surrey KT21 2HJ

The British Society of Experimental and Clinical Hypnosis
Department of Psychology
Middlewood Hospital
Sheffield S6 1TP

The United Kingdom Register of IBS Hypnotherapists
PO Box 57
Warrington WA5 1FG

Acupuncture

British Acupuncture Council
63 Jeddo Road
London W12 9HQ
Tel: 020 8735 0400
www.acupuncture.org.uk

British Medical Acupuncture Society
The Administrator, BMAS
12 Marbury House
Higher Whitley
Warrington
Cheshire WA4 4QW
Tel: 01925 730727
www.medical-acupuncture.co.uk

Alexander technique

The Society of Teachers of the Alexander Technique
1st Floor, Union House
39–51 Highgate Road
London NW5 1RS
Tel: 020 7284 3338
www.stat.org.uk

Aromatherapy

Aromatherapy Organisations Council
PO Box 19834
London SE25 6WF
Tel/Fax: 0870 7743477
www.oacuk.net

Aromatherapy and Allied Practitioners' Association
14 Orleans Road

Upper Norwood
London SE19 3TA
Tel/Fax: 020 8653 9152
www.aromatherapyuk.net

International Federation of Aromatherapists
182 Chiswick High Road
London W4 1PP
Tel: 020 8742 2605
www.int-fed-aromatherapy.co.uk

Ayurvedic medicine

Ayurvedic Medical Association UK
59 Dulverton Road
Selsdon
South Croydon
Surrey CR2 8PJ
Tel: 020 8657 6147
No website available.

Colonic irrigation

Association and Register of Colon Hydrotherapists
16 Drummond Ride
Tring
Herts HP23 5DE
Tel: 01442 827687
www.colonic-association.com

Herbal medicine (including oriental herbal medicine)

British Herbal Medicine Association
Sun House
Church Street
Stroud
Glos GL5 1JL
Tel: 01453 751402
www.bhma.info

European Herbal Practitioner Association
45a Corsica Street
London N5 1JT
Tel: 020 7354 5067
www.users.globalnet.co.uk/-ehpa

Register of Chinese Herbal Medicine
Tel: 0700 790332
www.rchm.co.uk

Homeopathy

British Homeopathic Association
15 Clerkenwell Close
London EC1R 0AA
Tel: 020 7566 7800
www.trusthomeopathy.org/trust

The Society of Homeopaths
4a Artizan Road
Northampton NN1 4HU
Tel: 01604 621400
www.homeopathy-soh.org

The UK Homoeopathic Medical Association
6 Livingstone Road
Gravesend
Kent DA12 5DZ
Tel: 01474 560336
www.homoeopathy.org

Kinesiology

Academy and Association of Systematic Kinesiology
39 Browns Road
Surbiton
Surrey KT5 8ST
Tel: 020 8399 3215

The Kinesiology Federation
PO Box 17153
Edinburgh EH11 3WQ
Tel: 08700 113545
www.kinesiologyfederation.org

Naturopathy

Association of Natural Medicine
19a Collingwood Road
Witham
Essex CM8 2DY
Tel: 01376 502762
www.anm.org.uk

Association of Physical and Natural Therapists
27 Old Gloucester Street
London WC1N 3XX
Tel: 07966 181588
www.apnt.org.uk

General Council and Register of Naturopaths
Goswell House
2 Goswell Road
Street
Somerset BA16 0JG
Tel: 08707 456984
www.naturopathy.org.uk

Polarity therapy

UK Polarity Therapy Association
Monomark House
27 Old Gloucester Street
London WC1N 3XX
Tel: 0700 7052748
www.ukpta.org.uk

Reflexology

Association of Reflexologists
27 Old Gloucester Street
London WC1N 3XX
Tel: 0870 5673320
www.aor.org.uk

British Reflexology Association
Administration Office
Monks Orchard
Whitbourne
Worcester WR6 5RB
Tel: 01886 821207
www.britreflex.co.uk

International Federation of Reflexologists
Croydon
Surrey CR0 1EF
Tel: 020 8667 9458
www.reflexology-ifr.com

Shiatsu

The Shiatsu Society
Eastlands Court
St Peter's Road
Rugby CV21 3QP
Tel: 0845 1304560
www.shiatsu.org

T'ai chi

T'ai Chi Union
1 Littlemill Drive
Balmoral Gardens
Crookston
Glasgow G53 7GE
Tel: 0141 810 3482
www.taichiunion.com

Yoga

The British Wheel of Yoga
25 Jermyn Street
Sleaford
Lincs NG34 7RU
Tel: 01529 306851
www.bwy.org.uk

General

British Complementary Medicine Association
PO Box 5122
Bournemouth BH8 0WG
www.bcma.co.uk

Complementary Healthcare Information Service
1 Kenworthy Street
Stalybridge
Cheshire SK15 2DX
Tel: 0161 339 2194
www.chisuk.org.uk

Complementary Medicine Association
Tel: 020 8305 9571
www.the-cma.org.uk

Guild of Complementary Practitioners
Liddell House
Liddell Close
Finchampstead
Berks RG40 4NS
Tel: 01189 735757
www.gcpnet.com

Books (besides this one)

Doctor, What's the Alternative? Dr Hilary Jones, Hodder & Stoughton, 1998 – an easy-read look at the benefits and limitations of both orthodox and alternative medicine and an appraisal, including a 'sceptic's view', of a whole range of complementary therapies. Not IBS-specific, however.

A Complete Guide to Relief from Irritable Bowel Syndrome, Christine P. Dancey and Susan Backhouse, Robinson Publishing, 1997 – edited by the founders of the self-help group, the IBS Network.

Websites

Although this information is as up-to-date as possible, it may be worth checking the web link for the most recent contact details before writing or phoning.

http://www.ibs-register – The UK register for therapists specialising in hypnosis for IBS.

www.babcp.com – The website of the British Association of Cognitive and Behavioural Psychotherapists. Extensive information on CBT including a 'find a therapist' search facility.

www.bps.org.uk – The British Psychological Society.

www.painsociety – The Pain Society is the representative body for all professionals involved in the management and understanding of pain.

www.nutrition.org.uk – The website of the British Nutrition Foundation.

www.studentbmj.com/back-issues – Information on IBS, food allergy and food intolerance.

www.foodsensitivity.com – Information on food sensitivity.

www.lactose.co.uk – Information on lactose intolerance.

www.candida-society.co.uk – Website for the National Candida Society.

www.surgerydoor.co.uk

www.rcgp.org.uk – Website for the Royal College of General Practitioners.

www.medicalcrossfire.com – Debates and insights in medicine.

www.nhsdirect.nhs.uk – Health information from the NHS.

www.netdoctor.co.uk – Website covering various diseases and conditions.

www.digestivedisorders.org.uk

www.altmedicine.about.com

www.the-cma.org.uk – Website of the Complementary Medical Association.

www.medical-acupuncture.co.uk

www.cyberspacehealthclinic.co.uk

www.aor.org.uk – Website of the Association of Reflexologists.

www.chisuk.org.uk – Complementary healthcare information service.

www.new-health.biz

www.chinese-remedy.co.uk – Website looking at Chinese herbal remedies.

www.mindbodydigestive.com – a US website with many well-written and informative articles on IBS

And good luck!

References

Bensoussan, A., Talley, N.J., Hing, M., Menzies, R., Guo, A. & Ngu, M. (1998) Treatment of irritable bowel syndrome with Chinese herbal medicine. *Journal of the American Medical Association*, **280**(18), 1585–1589.

Bischoff, S.C., Herrmann, A. & Manns, M.P. (1996) Prevalence of adverse reactions to food in patients with gastrointestinal disease. *Allergy*, **51**(11), 811–818.

Chalder, T., Darnley, S., Kennedy, T., Jones, R. & Wessely, S. (in press) A controlled trial of the addition of cognitive behavioural therapy to antispasmodic therapy for irritable bowel syndrome in primary care.

Chaudhary, N.A. & Truelove, S.C. (1962) The irritable colon syndrome. *Quarterly Journal of Medicine*, **31**(123), 307–322.

Dancey, C.P. & Backhouse, S. (eds) (1997) *A complete Guide to Relief from Irritable Bowel Syndrome*. London: Robinson.

Delvaux, M. (2001) Report on the Fourth International Symposium on Functional Gastrointestinal Disorders, March 30–April 2 2001, Milwaukee, Wisconsin; www.iffgd.org/symposium 2001.

Gershon, M. (1998) *The Second Brain*, HarperCollins, London.

Greene, B. & Blanchard, E.B. (1994) Cognitive therapy for irritable bowel syndrome. *Journal of Consulting and Clinical Psychology*, **62**, 576–582.

Guthrie, E., Creed, F., Dawson, D. & Tomenson, B. (1991) A controlled trial of psychological treatment for the irritable bowel syndrome. *Gastroenterology*, **100**, 450–457.

Heaton, K. & Thompson, W.G. (1999) *Fast Facts: Irritable Bowel Syndrome*. Lewisville, Tx: Health Press.

Highfield, R. (2001) *Daily Telegraph*, 10 August 2001.

Kellow, J.E., Phillips, S.F., Miller, L.J. & Zinsmeister, A.R. (1988) Dysmotility of the small intestine in irritable bowel syndrome. *Gut*, **29**(9), 1236–1243.

Klein, K.B. (1988) Controlled treatment trials in the irritable bowel syndrome, a critique. *Gastroenterology*, **95**, 232–241.

Kruis, W., Forstmaier, G., Scheurlen, C. & Stellaard, F. (1991) Effects of diets low and high in refined sugars on gut transit, bile acid metabolism and bacterial fermentation. *Gut*, **32**(4), 367–371.

Moore, A. (no date) You can conquer IBS. *Prevention Magazine* (US publication, no date); can be read on website www.byarden.com.

Nanda, R., James, R., Smith, H., Dudley, C.R. & Jewell, D.P. (1989) Food intolerance and irritable bowel syndrome. *Gut*, **30**(8), 1099–1104.

Read, N. (1997) Chapter 6 in Dancey, C. & Backhouse, S. (eds), *IBS: a Complete Guide to Relief from Irritable Bowel Syndrome*. London: Robinson, pp. 134–159.

Rumessen, J.J. & Gudmand-Hoyer, E. (1988) Functional bowel disease: malabsorption and abdominal distress after ingestion of fructose, sorbitol and fructose-sorbitol mixtures. *Gastroenterology*, **95**(3), 694–700.

Stefanini, G.F., Saggioro, A., Alvisi, V., Angelini, G., Capurso, L. & di Lorenzo, G. *et al.* (1995) Oral cromolyn sodium in comparison with elimination diet in the irritable bowel syndrome, diarrhoeic type. Multicenter study of 428 patients. *Scandinavian Journal of Gastroenterology*, **30**(6), 535–541.

Talbot, M. (2001) The placebo prescription. *New York Times Magazine*, January 9.

Thompson, W.G. (1989) *Gut Reactions: Understanding Symptoms of the Digestive Tract*. New York: Plenum Publishing.

Thompson, W.G., Longstreth, G.F., Drossman, D.A., Heaton, K.W., Irvine, E.J. & Muller-Lissner, S.A. (1999) Functional bowel disorders and functional abdominal pain. *Gut*, **45**(supp. II), 43–47.

Tovey, P. (2002) A single-blind trial of reflexology for irritable bowel. *British Journal of General Practice*, **52**, 19–23.

Vernia, P., Ricciardi, M.R., Frandina, C., Bilotta, T., Frieri, G. & Ital, J. (1995) Lactose malabsorption and irritable bowel syndrome: Effect of a long-term lactose-free diet. *Gastroenterology*, **27**(3), 117–121.

Whorwell, P.J., Prior, A. & Colgan, S.M. (1987) Hypnotherapy in severe irritable bowel syndrome: further experience. *Gut*, **28**, 423–452.

Whorwell, P.J., Prior, A. & Faragher, E.B. (1984) Controlled trial of hypnotherapy in the treatment of severe refractory irritable bowel syndrome. *Lancet*, **2**, 1232–1233.

Index

John Wiley & Sons
*publish a wide range of groundbreaking **books, journals** and **online resources** in many areas...*

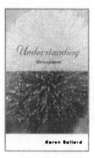
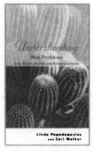
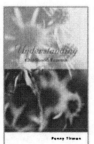

Lightning Source UK Ltd.
Milton Keynes UK
UKOW040412290312

189776UK00001B/25/P